Modern Concepts in Pancreatic Surgery

Editors

STEPHEN W. BEHRMAN
RONALD F. MARTIN

SURGICAL CLINICS
OF NORTH AMERICA

www.surgical.theclinics.com

Consulting Editor
RONALD F. MARTIN

June 2013 • Volume 93 • Number 3

ELSEVIER

1600 John F. Kennedy Boulevard • Suite 1800 • Philadelphia, Pennsylvania, 19103-2899

http://www.surgicaltheclinics.com

SURGICAL CLINICS OF NORTH AMERICA Volume 93, Number 3
June 2013 ISSN 0039-6109, ISBN-13: 978-1-4557-7335-0

Editor: John Vassallo, j.vassallo@elsevier.com

Developmental Editor: Teia Stone

Surgical Clinics of North America (ISSN 0039-6109) is published bimonthly by Elsevier Inc., 360 Park Avenue South, New York, NY 10010-1710. Months of publication are February, April, June, August, October, and December. Business and Editorial Offices: 1600 John F. Kennedy Blvd., Suite 1800, Philadelphia, PA 19103-2899. Periodicals postage paid at New York, NY and additional mailing offices. Subscription prices are $353.00 per year for US individuals, $598.00 per year for US institutions, $173.00 per year for US students and residents, $432.00 per year for Canadian individuals, $741.00 per year for Canadian institutions, $487.00 for international individuals, $741.00 per year for international institutions and $238.00 per year for Canadian and foreign students/residents. To receive student/resident rate, orders must be accompanied by name of affiliated institution, date of term, and the *signature* of program/residency coordinator on institution letterhead. Orders will be billed at individual rate until proof of status is received. Foreign air speed delivery is included in all *Clinics* subscription prices. All prices are subject to change without notice. POSTMASTER: Send address changes to *Surgical Clinics*, Elsevier Health Sciences Division, Subscription Customer Service, 3251 Riverport Lane, Maryland Heights, MO 63043. **Customer Service (orders, claims, online, change of address): Telephone: 1-800-654-2452 (U.S. and Canada); 314-447-8871 (outside U.S. and Canada). Fax: 314-447-8029. E-mail: journalscustomerservice-usa@elsevier.com (for print support); journalsonline support-usa@elsevier.com (for online support).**

Reprints. For copies of 100 or more, of articles in this publication, please contact the Commercial Reprints Department, Elsevier Inc., 360 Park Avenue South, New York, New York 10010-1710. Tel. (212) 633-3812, Fax: (212) 462-1935, e-mail: reprints@elsevier.com.

The Surgical Clinics of North America is also published in Spanish by McGraw-Hill Interamericana Editores S.A., P.O. Box 5-237 06500 Mexico D.F. Mexico; and in Portuguese by Interlivros Edicoes Ltda., Rua Comandante Coelho 1085, CEP 21250, Rio de Janeiro, Brazil; and in Greek by Paschalidis Medical Publications, Athens Greece.

The Surgical Clinics of North America is covered in *MEDLINE/PubMed (Index Medicus), EMBASE/Excerpta Medica, Current Contents/Clinical Medicine, Current Contents/Life Sciences, Science Citation Index,* and *ISI/BIOMED.*

Printed and bound by CPI Group (UK) Ltd, Croydon, CR0 4YY

Transferred to digital print 2013

Contributors

CONSULTING EDITOR

RONALD F. MARTIN, MD, FACS
Staff Surgeon, Department of Surgery, Marshfield Clinic, Marshfield, Wisconsin; Clinical, Associate Professor, University of Wisconsin School of Medicine and Public Health, Madison, Wisconsin; Colonel, Medical Corps, United States Army Reserve

EDITORS

STEPHEN W. BEHRMAN, MD, FACS
Professor of Surgery, Division of Surgical Oncology, Department of Surgery, University of Tennessee Health Science Center, Memphis, Tennessee

RONALD F. MARTIN, MD, FACS
Staff Surgeon, Department of Surgery, Marshfield Clinic, Marshfield, Wisconsin; Clinical, Associate Professor, University of Wisconsin School of Medicine and Public Health, Madison, Wisconsin; Colonel, Medical Corps, United States Army Reserve

AUTHORS

MICHAEL H. BAHR, MD
Department of Surgery, University of Louisville School of Medicine, Louisville, Kentucky

PETER A. BANKS, MD
Professor of Medicine, Division of Gastroenterology, Hepatology and Endoscopy, Brigham and Women's Hospital, Harvard Medical School, Boston, Massachusetts

STEPHEN W. BEHRMAN, MD, FACS
Professor of Surgery, Division of Surgical Oncology, Department of Surgery, University of Tennessee Health Science Center, Memphis, Tennessee

JEFFREY A. BLATNIK, MD
Department of Surgery, University Hospitals Case Medical Center, Case Western Reserve University, Cleveland, Ohio

THOMAS L. BOLLEN, MD
Department of Radiology, St. Antonius Hospital, Nieuwegein, The Netherlands

TERESA A. BRENTNALL, MD
Professor, Department of Gastroenterology, Digestive Diseases Center, University of Washington, Seattle, Washington

JOHN D. CHRISTEIN, MD
Associate Professor, Department of Surgery, The Kirklin Clinic, UAB Medical Center, Birmingham, Alabama

YUN SHIN CHUN, MD
Assistant Professor, Department of Surgical Oncology, Fox Chase Cancer Center, Philadelphia, Pennsylvania

BRIAN R. DAVIS, MD, FACS
Assistant Professor, Department of Surgery, Texas Tech University Health Sciences Center at El Paso, El Paso, Texas

CHRISTOS DERVENIS, MD
1st Department of Surgery, Agia Olga Hospital, Athens, Greece

PAXTON V. DICKSON, MD
Assistant Professor of Surgery, Division of Surgical Oncology, Department of Surgery, University of Tennessee Health Science Center, Memphis, Tennessee

WILLIAM E. FISHER, MD, FACS
Professor, Michael E. DeBakey Department of Surgery; Director, Elkins Pancreas Center, Baylor College of Medicine, Houston, Texas

HEIN G. GOOSZEN, MD
Professor and Chair, Evidence-Based Surgery Research Unit, University of Nijmegen, Nijmegen, The Netherlands

JEFFREY M. HARDACRE, MD, FACS
Associate Professor, Department of Surgery, University Hospitals Case Medical Center, Case Western Reserve University, Cleveland, Ohio

AMANDA R. HEIN, MD
Resident in General Surgery, Department of General Surgery, Marshfield Clinics and Saint Joseph's Hospital, Marshfield, Wisconsin

JOHN P. HOFFMAN, MD, FACS
Chief, Pancreaticobiliary Service, Department of Surgical Oncology, Fox Chase Cancer Center, Philadelphia, Pennsylvania

THOMAS J. HOWARD, MD, FACS
Professor, Hepatobiliary Surgical Cancer Care, Community Hospital North, Indianapolis, Indiana

COLIN D. JOHNSON, MChir, FRCS
University Surgical Unit, Southampton General Hospital, Southampton, United Kingdom

RONALD F. MARTIN, MD, FACS
Staff Surgeon, Department of Surgery, Marshfield Clinic, Marshfield, Wisconsin; Clinical, Associate Professor, University of Wisconsin School of Medicine and Public Health, Madison, Wisconsin; Colonel, Medical Corps, United States Army Reserve

JOHN C. McAULIFFE, MD, PhD
Department of Surgery, The Kirklin Clinic, UAB Medical Center, Birmingham, Alabama

SOMALA MOHAMMED, MD
General Surgery Resident, Division of General Surgery, Michael E. DeBakey Department of Surgery; Elkins Pancreas Center, Baylor College of Medicine, Houston, Texas

PAVLOS PAPAVASILIOU, MD
Texas Oncology Surgical Specialists, Baylor Sammons Cancer Center; Department of Surgery, Baylor University Medical Center, Dallas, Texas

MICHAEL G. SARR, MD, FACS
Professor of Surgery, Department of Surgery, Mayo Clinic, Rochester, Minnesota

ADAM W. TEMPLETON, MD
Senior Fellow, Department of Gastroenterology, Digestive Diseases Center, University of Washington, Seattle, Washington

GREGORY G. TSIOTOS, MD
Division of Digestive Surgery, Metropolitan Hospital, Athens, Greece

SANTHI SWAROOP VEGE, MD
Professor of Medicine, Director, Pancreas Group, Division of Gastroenterology and Hepatology, Department of Medicine, Mayo Clinic, Rochester, Minnesota

CAROLINE S. VERBEKE, MD, PhD, FRCPath
Division of Pathology, Department of Laboratory Medicine, Karolinska Institute, Karolinska University Hospital, Stockholm, Sweden

GARY C. VITALE, MD, FACS
Professor, Department of Surgery, University of Louisville School of Medicine, Louisville, Kentucky

CHARLES M. VOLLMER Jr, MD, FACS
Director of Pancreatic Surgery, Associate Professor of Surgery, Department of Surgery, Hospital of the University of Pennsylvania, University of Pennsylvania School of Medicine, Philadelphia, Pennsylvania

MICHAEL G. SARR, MD, FACS
Professor of Surgery, Department of Surgery, Mayo Clinic, Rochester, Minnesota

ADAM W. EMBLETON, MD
Senior Fellow, Department of Gastroenterology, Digestive Diseases Center, University of Washington, Seattle, Washington

GREGORY G. TSIOTOS, MD
Division of Digestive Surgery, Metropolitan Hospital, Athens, Greece

SANTHI SWAROOP VEGE, MD
Professor of Medicine, Director, Pancreas Group, Division of Gastroenterology and Hepatology, Department of Medicine, Mayo Clinic, Rochester, Minnesota

CAROLINE S. VERBEKE, MD, PhD, FRCPath
Division of Pathology, Department of Laboratory Medicine, Karolinska Institute, Karolinska University Hospital, Stockholm, Sweden

GARY C. VITALE, MD, FACS
Professor, Department of Surgery, University of Louisville School of Medicine, Louisville, Kentucky

CHARLES M. VOLLMER Jr, MD, FACS
Director of Pancreatic Surgery, Associate Professor of Surgery, Department of Surgery, Hospital of the University of Pennsylvania, University of Pennsylvania School of Medicine, Philadelphia, Pennsylvania

Contents

This study aims to update the 1991 Atlanta Classification of acute pancreatitis, to standardize the reporting of and terminology of the disease and its complications. Important features of this classification have incorporated new insights into the disease learned over the last 20 years, including the recognition that acute pancreatitis and its complications involve a dynamic process involving two phases, early and late. The accurate and consistent description of acute pancreatitis will help to improve the stratification and reporting of new methods of care of acute pancreatitis across different practices, geographic areas, and countries.

Patients presenting with acute pancreatitis can be complex on different levels. Having a multifaceted approach to these patients is often necessary with radiographic, endoscopic, and surgical modalities all working to benefit the patient. Major surgical intervention can often be avoided or augmented by therapeutic and diagnostic endoscopic maneuvers. The diagnostic role of endoscopy in patients presenting with acute idiopathic pancreatitis can help define specific causative factors and ameliorate symptoms by endoscopic maneuvers. Etiologies of an acute pancreatitis episode, such as choledocholithiasis with or without concomitant cholangitis, microlithiasis or biliary sludge, and anatomic anomalies, such as pancreas divisum and pancreatobiliary ductal anomalies, often improve after endoscopic therapy.

The role of antimicrobial therapy in patients with severe acute pancreatitis is to treat secondary pancreatic infections to prevent systemic sepsis and death. Infected pancreatic necrosis is diagnosed using image-directed fine needle aspiration with culture and Gram's stain. Prophylactic antibiotics have not proven efficacious, while the precise timely detection of secondary pancreatic infections is often elusive. A high clinical index of suspicion should prompt the empiric initiation of antimicrobial therapy until culture results are available. Positive cultures should guide antimicrobial therapy, and for infected pancreatic necrosis, antibiotics should be used in conjunction with interventional techniques for source control.

R1 rate and the prognostic significance of margin involvement. This article discusses the current lack of consensus regarding the definition and diagnostic criteria of R1 resection, the terminology for the various surgical margins, and the pathology grossing technique. Recent developments in pathology examination that allow a more accurate margin assessment are described. Furthermore, the need of a quality assurance system that ensures robustness and comparability of data on resection margins in pancreatic cancer is highlighted.

Historically, borderline resectable (BLR) pancreatic cancer has had many definitions, which has made interpretation of treatment data and outcomes difficult. Advances in imaging, surgical technique, and the potential benefit of neoadjuvant therapy have emphasized the need for uniform classification. Despite recent efforts to provide a clearer definition, prospective randomized trials are lacking in the literature. This article reviews current definitions, treatment sequences, outcomes, and prognostic factors associated with BLR pancreatic cancer. Further clarification and consensus on the definition of BLR pancreatic cancer will allow for further data collection and cooperation in future efforts to make progress and standardize treatment.

Pancreatic neuroendocrine tumors account for 1% to 2% of pancreatic neoplasms and may occur sporadically or as part of a hereditary syndrome. Patients may present with symptoms related to hormone secretion by functional tumors or to locally advanced or metastatic nonfunctional tumors. Asymptomatic pancreatic neuroendocrine tumors are increasingly detected incidentally during abdominal imaging performed for other reasons. The management of localized pancreatic neuroendocrine tumors is surgical resection. Hepatic metastases are common and their management involves a variety of liver-directed therapies, which should be tailored according to extent of disease, symptoms, presence of extrahepatic metastases, and patient performance status.

As the practice of pancreatic surgery evolves to encompass a wider array of clinical indications, incorporate increasingly complex technologies, and provide care to an aging population with many comorbid conditions, systematic assessment of quality and outcomes in an effort to improve the quality of care is imperative. This article discusses the volume-outcomes relationship that exists in pancreatic surgery, trends in centralization of practice within the field, common outcomes measures, and the complexity of assessing quality metrics. It also highlights surgical outcomes from several high-volume institutions and recent developments in quality metrics within pancreatic surgery.

Pancreas surgery is a paradigm for high-acuity surgical specialization. Given the current intrigue over containing health care expenditures, pancreas surgery provides an ideal model to investigate the cost of care. This article explores the economics of this field from literature accrued over the last 2 decades. The cost of performing a pancreatic resection is established and then embellished with a discussion of the effects of clinical care paths. Then the influence of complications on costs is explored. Next, cost is investigated as an emerging outcome metric regarding variations in pancreatic surgical care. Finally, the societal-level fiscal impact is considered.

SURGICAL CLINICS OF NORTH AMERICA

FORTHCOMING ISSUES

August 2013
Vascular Surgery and Endovascular Therapy
Girma Tefera, MD, *Editor*

October 2013
Abdominal Wall Reconstruction
Michael Rosen, MD, *Editor*

December 2013
Acute Care Surgery
George Velmahos, MD, *Editor*

RECENT ISSUES

April 2013
Multidisciplinary Breast Management
George M. Fuhrman, MD, and
Tari A. King, MD, *Editors*

February 2013
**Complications, Considerations and
Consequences of Colorectal Surgery**
Scott R. Steele, MD, *Editor*

December 2012
Surgical Critical Care
John A. Weigelt, MD, *Editor*

October 2012
**Contemporary Management of Esophageal
Malignancy**
Chadrick E. Denlinger, MD, and
Carolyn E. Reed, MD, *Editors*

ISSUE OF RELATED INTEREST

Surgical Oncology Clinics of North America April 2010 (Vol. 19, Issue 2)
Pancreatic Cancer: Current Concepts in Treatment and Research
Andrew M. Lowy, MD, FACS, *Editor*

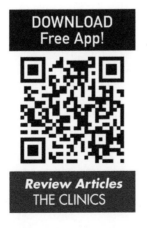

**DOWNLOAD
Free App!**

Review Articles
THE CLINICS

NOW AVAILABLE FOR YOUR iPhone and iPad

Foreword

Modern Concepts in Pancreatic Surgery

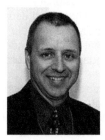

Ronald F. Martin, MD, FACS
Consulting Editor

I have always found the contradictions in our behaviors more interesting than the consistencies. For example, surgeons as a group tend to be fiercely autonomous in their attitudes and desires, yet they tend to train and work in groups. In my opinion, they work more effectively in group collaborations than when working alone.

There has been a long tradition of individual achievement in surgery. Most of the people who were my mentors grew up in the days of the "One riot, one ranger" mentality and regaled us of stories of wooden ships and iron men. Every surgeon worth his salt was on call every day and every night and every surgeon was captain of the ship.

Well, the images of those days have pretty well faded in the rear view mirror. Not only are we not necessarily captains of the ships but also it is not even clear to me that we are on ships. In an average work day after reviewing images read at night by "partners" living in Hawaii, one may render a consultation via telehealth to a gastroenterologist colleague working in another town altogether. In my world, at least, gone are the days of consulting about a problem to a patient's primary care physician who would then either manage the patient or turn her briefly over to us for operative intervention and perioperative care. Today, I try to find who is job sharing with the primary care provider to let them know that a whole series of consultants are now engaged in the care of the patient. More often than not, the reply I get is, "Okay, um, thanks. Let me know how Mr Jones does." The phone is usually back on the hook before I can say, "Actually, her name is Mrs Smith...." To say that care has become frequently decentralized and even fragmented would be a bit of an understatement.

There are probably many reasons for this change: some of it is a simple response to the increasing complexity of paperwork (which is now electronic); some of it is due to hyperspecialization, and some of it may be due to collective "burnout." Yet, I think there may be a more structural issue that accounts for these changes—the shifting balance between individual and collective responsibility. When I started in surgical practice I was in a solo private practice model. We all were. Yet, ironically, I sometimes think

Surg Clin N Am 93 (2013) xiii–xiv
http://dx.doi.org/10.1016/j.suc.2013.04.001
0039-6109/13/$ – see front matter © 2013 Published by Elsevier Inc.

surgical.theclinics.com

we worked more closely and communicated more readily then than we do now. Everybody knew that if you were caring for a patient you had to tie up all the loose ends yourself; perhaps because you couldn't blame anyone else if something came unraveled.

Today, I work in a system that is extremely connected via digital means and people rarely directly communicate with one another. Instead of phone calls, I get e-mails that hyperlink me to notes and texts. Most often I have to divine what the question or reason for getting the text or e-mail is from reading the record. Occasionally, I get it right. When something falls through the cracks now, there is a diffuse and usually impenetrable layer that obscures who—if anybody—was actually responsible for what went wrong. I would agree that the majority of advances that we have made in the digital era are truly advances, but we have lost some really fundamental processes that were cheap, effective, and frequently educational.

We surgeons and physicians are not alone in these issues. Much of the contentious national political discord boils down to disagreements over individual versus collective responsibility and reward. In the extreme, the individualists think they built everything themselves in some sort of vacuum and the collectivists seem to think that they deserve a cut of what everybody else has just for showing up on the planet. Neither side seems to be willing to move toward the center. Some people feel strongly that they are more productive working at home in isolation, while other people feel that people are more productive being co-located. Both sides again are probably right for varying circumstances. Productivity alone may be more readily decentralized, whereas innovation probably requires greater in-person random interaction—the water-cooler effect. Again, the right solution depends on the problem being solved.

Being Consulting Editor of the *Surgical Clinics of North America* has been a fascinating experience for many reasons. The one thing that continues to amaze me every 2 months is just how effectively people with wildly different practices and very different pressures come together to produce such high-quality work. Almost all of the contributors to these issues are extremely busy and dedicated clinicians, yet they unfailingly make time and find ways to contribute to these collective projects with little to gain for their efforts other than the satisfaction of helping the team turn out good work. If I could always find that enthusiasm and effort in my clinical practice, it would be life altering.

Dr Behrman and I have been fortunate to be able to turn to our closest brethren to produce this issue on pancreatic surgery. We are deeply indebted to all who contributed. I am particularly indebted to Dr Steve Behrman not just for carrying more than his share of the load, as he always does, but also for many, many years of enduring friendship. He is one of those people who I can always call day or night and know he is there to help.

I hope the reader of this issue not only finds knowledge and guidance in the management of pancreatic disorders but also takes stock in what can be done when we focus a bit more on what we can do collectively and a bit less on what doesn't seem like it is our specific responsibility. A little selflessness can be very self-rewarding.

Ronald F. Martin, MD, FACS
Department of Surgery
Marshfield Clinic
1000 North Oak Avenue
Marshfield, WI 54449, USA

E-mail address:
martin.ronald@marshfieldclinic.org

Preface

Modern Concepts in Pancreatic Surgery

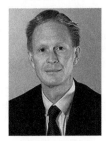
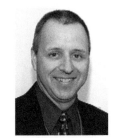

Stephen W. Behrman, MD, FACS   Ronald F. Martin, MD, FACS
Editors

Our knowledge of pancreatic diseases continues to evolve rapidly, yet often we feel defeated when dealing with the individual patient. Countless times we approach pancreatic pathology with confidence only to find that this fickle organ has once again thrown us a knuckleball—patients too often on the losing end, and defeat that we all find intolerable. Perhaps that's what drives those of us that have the temerity to not only operate on these patients but also offer them hope as well. I would submit that progress is being made, perhaps not fast enough, but we are seeing success little by little. Multi-institutional collaboration has been particularly helpful in this regard, and it is reassuring to know that pancreatic surgeons are working collectively to further advance our understanding of both benign and malignant pancreatic disorders. Such efforts by pancreatic specialists allow close scrutiny of surgical outcomes and quality metrics that engender optimal patient care.

Ron Martin and I are pleased to offer this update on the surgical management of pancreatic disorders. Rather than focus on one specific area of pancreatic pathology, we sought to broaden the scope of this compendium to a spectrum of topics relevant to all physicians and surgeons that treat those afflicted with diseases of the pancreas. Thus, this issue of the *Surgical Clinics of North America* offers a timely and authoritative treatise that will not only educate but also hopefully prosper future research endeavors.

We are indebted to our coauthors for their contributions in their individual fields of expertise. All are respected, busy clinicians that practice their craft to the highest level.

Surg Clin N Am 93 (2013) xv–xvi
http://dx.doi.org/10.1016/j.suc.2013.03.001
0039-6109/13/$ – see front matter © 2013 Published by Elsevier Inc.

surgical.theclinics.com

Their time and commitment to this monograph in the face of other demands is deeply appreciated and we know you will find their work stimulating and a joy to read.

Stephen W. Behrman, MD, FACS
Division of Surgical Oncology
Department of Surgery
University of Tennessee Health Science Center
910 Madison Avenue
Suite 208
Memphis, TN 38163, USA

Ronald F. Martin, MD, FACS
Department of Surgery
Marshfield Clinic
1000 North Oak Avenue
Marshfield, WI 54449, USA

E-mail addresses:
sbehrman@uthsc.edu (S.W. Behrman)
martin.ronald@marshfieldclinic.org (R.F. Martin)

The New Revised Classification of Acute Pancreatitis 2012

Michael G. Sarr, MD[a],*, Peter A. Banks, MD[b],
Thomas L. Bollen, MD[c], Christos Dervenis, MD[d],
Hein G. Gooszen, MD[e], Colin D. Johnson, MChir, FRCS[f],
Gregory G. Tsiotos, MD[g], Santhi Swaroop Vege, MD[h]

KEYWORDS

- Classification • Acute pancreatitis • Interstitial edematous pancreatitis
- Necrotizing pancreatitis

KEY POINTS

- The aim of this study is to update the original 1991 Atlanta Classification of acute pancreatitis to standardize the reporting of and terminology of the disease and its complications.
- Important features of this classification have incorporated the new insights into the disease learned over the last 20 years, including the recognition that acute pancreatitis and its complications involve a dynamic process involving two phases, early and late.
- The accurate and consistent description of the two types of acute pancreatitis (interstitial edematous pancreatitis and necrotizing pancreatitis), its severity, and, possibly most importantly, the description of local complications based on characteristics of fluid and necrosis involving the peripancreatic collections, will help to improve the stratification and reporting of new methods of care of acute pancreatitis across different practices, geographic areas, and countries.
- By using a common terminology, the advancement of the science of acute pancreatitis should be facilitated.

INTRODUCTION

More than 20 years have passed since the first concerted effort to classify acute pancreatitis by the Atlanta Classification, spearheaded by Edward Bradley in 1991.[1] At the time, this classification was an attempt to define a common terminology and

[a] Department of Surgery, Mayo Clinic (GU 10-01), 200 First Street Southwest, Rochester, MN 55905, USA; [b] Division of Gastroenterology, Hepatology and Endoscopy, Brigham and Women's Hospital, Harvard Medical School, Boston, MA, USA; [c] Department of Radiology, St Antonius Hospital, Nieuwegein, The Netherlands; [d] 1st Department of Surgery, Agia Olga Hospital, Athens, Greece; [e] Evidence-Based Surgery Research Unit, University of Nijmegen, Nijmegen, The Netherlands; [f] University Surgical Unit, Southampton General Hospital, Southampton, UK; [g] Division of Digestive Surgery, Metropolitan Hospital, Athens, Greece; [h] Pancreas Group, Division of Gastroenterology and Hepatology, Department of Medicine, Mayo Clinic, Rochester, MN, USA
* Corresponding author.
E-mail address: sarr.michael@mayo.edu

Surg Clin N Am 93 (2013) 549–562
http://dx.doi.org/10.1016/j.suc.2013.02.012
0039-6109/13/$ – see front matter © 2013 Elsevier Inc. All rights reserved.

define the severity of the disease such that physicians around the world would accept and adopt a uniform classification. Although novel at the time, the classification defined and used several terms that never "caught on," and the actual classification as written by the Atlanta Conference, while referred to by many articles, has not been accepted or used universally.[2] Moreover, in these last 20 years our understanding of the etiopathogenesis of acute pancreatitis, its natural history, the various markers of severity, and, equally important, the features of the disease on state-of-the-art cross-sectional imaging, have led to a plethora of often confusing and imprecisely used terms. Indeed, a common terminology for the disease, its severity, and, possibly most importantly, the pancreatic and peripancreatic "fluid" collections, have yet to be acknowledged and adopted. Because of this confusion, a group of researchers decided to revise the Atlanta Classification using a new technique for a global, Web-based "virtual" consensus conference over the Internet. Although the concept was novel, the idea of a Web-based global consensus, as described in this article, was only partially successful. Nevertheless, using this approach initially, with very helpful and insightful input from numerous pancreatologists of many different disciplines (gastroenterology, surgery, pathology, diagnostic and interventional radiology, gastrointestinal endoscopy, and acute care medicine/surgery) around the world, a new classification was developed and vetted through many different international societies dealing with acute pancreatitis. Using this input, the Working Group (the authors of this article) then collated the evidence-based literature whenever available to construct a new classification, in part based on the two phases of the natural history of the disease (the first week or two, and the next several weeks/months that follow). The product of the past 5 years of work culminated in the Classification of Acute Pancreatitis 2012.[3] This classification addresses diagnosis, types of acute pancreatitis, severity, and definition of pancreatic and peripancreatic collections, which are discussed herein. The authors hope that this classification will unify the terminology to allow global consensus and facilitate comparison of studies published in the literature.

DIAGNOSIS OF ACUTE PANCREATITIS

The diagnosis of this disease is usually straightforward and, as described in many studies, involves a combination of symptoms, physical examination, and focused laboratory values. This classification requires 2 of the following 3 features: (1) central upper abdominal pain usually of acute onset often radiating through to the back; (2) serum amylase or lipase activity greater than 3 times the upper limit of normal; and (3) characteristic features on cross-sectional abdominal imaging consistent with the diagnosis of acute pancreatitis (see later discussion). Note that not every patient requires pancreatic imaging; for instance, for the patient with characteristic abdominal pain and increased serum amylase/lipase activity, a contrast-enhanced computed tomography (CECT) or magnetic resonance imaging (MRI) is usually not required on admission or later (if it is mild acute pancreatitis), provided the clinical picture is that of acute pancreatitis.

DEFINITION OF THE TWO TYPES OF ACUTE PANCREATITIS

There are two basically different forms of acute pancreatitis: interstitial edematous pancreatitis and necrotizing pancreatitis.

Interstitial Edematous Pancreatitis

The majority (80%–90%) of patients presenting with the clinical picture of acute pancreatitis will have this more mild form. The differentiating characteristic of acute interstitial edematous pancreatitis is the lack of pancreatic parenchymal necrosis or peripancreatic necrosis evident on imaging. The associated findings are usually diffuse (or, on occasion, localized) enlargement of the pancreas secondary to inflammatory edema (**Fig. 1**); there may also be some peripancreatic fluid (see the section on pancreatic and peripancreatic collections). The pancreatic parenchyma and surrounding tissues may have haziness and stranding secondary to inflammatory edema, but there is no necrosis evident on cross-sectional imaging. The clinical picture of this form of acute pancreatitis usually resolves quickly over the first week.

Necrotizing Pancreatitis

The hallmark of this form of acute pancreatitis is the presence of tissue necrosis, either of the pancreatic parenchyma or the peripancreatic tissues. Necrotizing pancreatitis most commonly involves both the pancreatic parenchyma and the peripancreatic tissue (**Fig. 2**) or the peripancreatic tissue alone (**Fig. 3**); rarely, the necrosis is limited only to the pancreatic parenchyma. Therefore, necrotizing pancreatitis is classified as pancreatic parenchymal necrosis alone, pancreatic parenchymal and peripancreatic necrosis, or peripancreatic necrosis alone. Involvement of the pancreatic parenchyma usually heralds a disease more severe than peripancreatic necrosis alone.[4,5]

Early in the illness (during the first week), the differentiation of "necrosis" can be difficult on CECT. For the pancreatic parenchyma, nonperfusion of the pancreatic gland is usually evident. For the peripancreatic region, obvious loss of "perfusion" of the retroperitoneal fat is not evident (this area has little radiographic "perfusion" even normally), and the diagnosis of necrosis is usually made based on the presence of local inflammatory changes and some element of associated fluid, but also a solid component (see later discussion). Recognition of this peripancreatic necrosis is difficult during the first week of the disease, but thereafter the diagnosis on imaging becomes more apparent, with a more heterogeneous collection of both solid and liquid components.

Infected Versus Sterile Necrosis

Necrotizing pancreatitis should also be labeled either infected or sterile. Infection is rare during the first week.[6,7] Infection can be diagnosed based on ongoing signs of sepsis

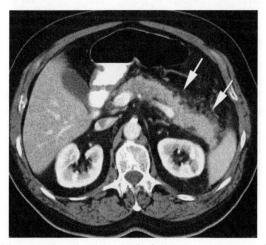

Fig. 1. A 48-year-old man with acute interstitial edematous pancreatitis. There is peripancreatic fat stranding (*arrows*); the pancreas enhances completely.

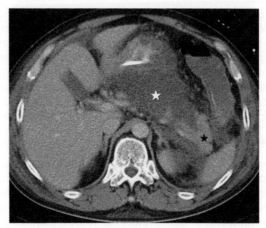

Fig. 2. A 39-year-old woman with acute necrotizing pancreatitis. There is extensive nonenhancement representing parenchymal necrosis (*white star*) of the body of the pancreas. Part of the pancreatic tail shows normal enhancement (*black star*).

and/or the combination of clinical signs and the computed tomographic imaging when extraluminal gas is present within areas of necrosis in the pancreatic and/or peripancreatic tissues (**Fig. 4**). Similarly, the diagnosis of infected necrosis can be made based on percutaneous, image-guided fine-needle aspiration when bacteria and/or fungi are seen on Gram stain and the culture is positive. Lack of positive Gram stain or culture positivity should be interpreted with some caution. The presence of suppuration (numerous polymorphonuclear cells) is somewhat variable; the longer the duration of the infection, the more suppuration. Infection may also be diagnosed as a secondary event after instrumentation of whatever form (percutaneous, endoscopic, operative); secondary infection is associated with increased mortality and morbidity.[8]

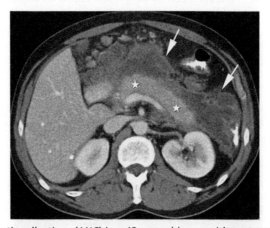

Fig. 3. Acute necrotic collections (ANC) in a 42-year-old man with acute necrotizing pancreatitis involving only the peripancreatic tissues. Note normal enhancement of the entire pancreatic parenchyma (*white stars*) and the heterogeneous, nonliquid peripancreatic components in the retroperitoneum and mesentery of the transverse mesocolon (*white arrows* pointing at the borders of the ANC).

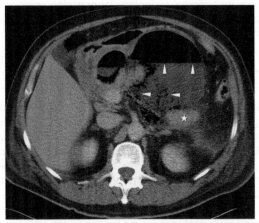

Fig. 4. A 45-year-old man with acute necrotizing pancreatitis complicated by infected pancreatic necrosis. The pancreatic tail (*white star*) enhances normally. There is a large heterogeneous ANC in the pancreatic and peripancreatic area with presence of impacted gas bubbles (*horizontal white arrowheads*) and gas-fluid level (*vertical white arrowheads*), usually a sign of infection of the necrosis.

SEVERITY OF THE DISEASE

Classifying the severity of the disease is important when comparing different institutional experiences, talking with patients about prognosis, planning therapy, and comparing new methods of management.

This classification of severity of acute pancreatitis defines 3 degrees of severity: mild acute pancreatitis, moderately severe acute pancreatitis, and severe acute pancreatitis. These levels of severity are based on the presence and/or absence of persistent organ failure and local and systemic complications (see later discussion). In general, mild acute pancreatitis resolves within several days to a week, moderately severe acute pancreatitis resolves slowly and may require interventions, and severe acute pancreatitis, in addition to longer hospital stay and interventions, is also associated with organ failure and death.

Definition of Organ Failure (Persistent or Transient)

Persistent organ failure for at least 48 hours has proved to be the most reliable marker for disease severity in acute pancreatitis.[9,10] Organ failure has been scored by many different systems, and numerous serum markers have also been evaluated. After careful review of the literature as well as consideration of the pathogenesis and the course of acute pancreatitis, the authors chose the modified Marshall scoring system.[11] This scoring system is easy and universally applicable because it does not require any sophisticated assays or monitoring and, most importantly, stratifies disease severity objectively and easily.[12] This scoring system targets the 3 organ systems most commonly affected by the systemic inflammatory response syndrome (SIRS) that accompanies severe acute pancreatitis: respiratory, cardiovascular, and renal (**Table 1**). Persistent organ failure is defined as a score of 2 or more for more than 48 hours for 1 (or more) of the 3 organ systems using the modified Marshall scoring system. By contrast, transient organ failure is a score of 2 or more, but for less than 48 hours. This scoring system is preferred over the Sepsis-related Organ Failure Assessment (SOFA) system,[13] which is used for patients in a critical care unit and also takes into

Table 1
Modified Marshall scoring system

Organ System	Score				
	0	1	2	3	4
Respiratory (Pao$_2$/Fio$_2$)	>400	301–400	201–300	101–200	≤101
Renal[a]					
Serum creatinine, μmol/L	≤134	134–169	170–310	311–439	>439
Serum creatinine, mg/dL	<1.4	1.4–1.8	1.9–3.6	3.6–4.9	>4.9
Cardiovascular (systolic blood pressure, mm Hg)[b]	>90	<90 Fluid responsive	<90 Not fluid responsive	<90, pH <7.3	<90, pH <7.2

A score of 2 or more in any system defines the presence of organ failure.

[a] Scoring patients with preexistent chronic renal failure depends on the extent of deterioration over baseline renal function. Calculations for a baseline serum creatinine ≥134 μmol/L or ≥1.4 mg/dL are not available.

[b] Off inotropic support.

Modified from Banks PA, Bollen TL, Dervenis C, et al. Classification of acute pancreatitis—2012: revision of the Atlanta Classification and Definitions by International Consensus. Gut 2013;62;102–11.

consideration other criteria. The modified Marshall scoring system can be used repeatedly, both early and late in the course of the disease, to classify severity.

Definition of Local Complications

Unlike in the prior 1991 Atlanta Classification, the natural history, clinical consequences, and, most importantly, the definition of pancreatic and peripancreatic collections are now better understood. Local complications in the current 2012 classification include acute peripancreatic fluid collections, pancreatic pseudocysts, acute necrotic collections, and walled-off necrosis (see later discussion). Other local complications include splenic/portal vein thrombosis, colonic necrosis, retroperitoneal hemorrhage, and gastric outlet dysfunction. One might think of the local complications as those that delay hospital discharge or require intervention but do not necessarily cause death. Of course, one would expect the presence of a local complication by persistence of abdominal pain, secondary increases in serum amylase/lipase activity, organ failure, fever/chills, and so forth. Such symptoms usually prompt a cross-sectional imaging procedure to search for these complications.

Definition of Systemic Complications

These systemic complications involve de novo occurrence of renal, circulatory, or respiratory organ failure or exacerbation of serious preexisting comorbidities related directly to the acute pancreatitis. Examples of these comorbidities include coronary artery disease, congestive heart failure, chronic obstructive lung disease, diabetes, and chronic liver disease. Note that organ failure as defined by the modified Marshall score is not considered as part of these systemic complications, and a distinction is made between persistent organ failure (a sign of severe acute pancreatitis; see later discussion) and systemic complications. These complications result from the systemic inflammatory response to acute pancreatitis, and may be further exacerbated by the need for fluid resuscitation.

Phases of Acute Pancreatitis

In general there are two phases of this dynamic disease of acute pancreatitis, which overlap one another: the early phase, which usually lasts only 1 week or so, and the late phase, which can persist for weeks to months.

During the early phase, most of the systemic manifestations of the disease are a consequence of the host response to the pancreatic injury. This early phase is secondary to the cytokine cascade, which manifests as SIRS,[14] and/or the compensatory anti-inflammatory syndrome (CARS), which can predispose to infection.[15] When SIRS or CARS persist, organ failure becomes much more likely. The determinant of the severity of the acute pancreatitis is primarily the presence and duration of organ failure: transient organ failure (<48 hours' duration) and persistent organ failure (>48 hours' duration). If the organ failure involves more than 1 organ, the terms multiple organ failure or multiple organ dysfunction syndrome are appropriate.

The late phase of acute pancreatitis is characterized by the persistence of systemic signs of ongoing inflammation, by the presence of local and systemic complications, and/or by transient or persistent organ failure. By definition, the late phase occurs only in patients with moderately severe or severe acute pancreatitis.

Definition of Severity of Acute Pancreatitis

The need to define severity is important for several reasons. It is important to identify patients on admission or during the first 24 to 48 hours who will require aggressive resuscitation/treatment, either so they are monitored closely in an intensive care unit or so they can be transferred to a high-acuity care hospital. The definition of severity will not be able to be made definitively in the first 48 hours; therefore, patients with SIRS should be treated as if they have severe acute pancreatitis. Second, such stratification allows various practices around the world to compare treatments and experiences in a more objective scoring/classification system.

This classification defines 3 degrees of severity: mild, moderately severe, and severe acute pancreatitis (**Box 1**). These degrees of severity separate patients well into 3 groups according to the morbidity and mortality of the disease.

Mild Acute Pancreatitis

Mild acute pancreatitis is defined as acute pancreatitis without organ failure or local or systemic complications. These patients resolve their symptoms rapidly and are

---

Box 1
Degrees of severity

Mild Acute Pancreatitis

- No organ failure
- Lack of local or systemic complications

Moderately Severe Acute Pancreatitis

- Organ failure that resolves within 48 hours (transient organ failure) and/or
- Local or systemic complications (sterile or infected) without persistent organ failure

Severe Acute Pancreatitis

- Persistent single or multiple organ failure (>48 hours)

Modified from Banks PA, Bollen TL, Dervenis C, et al. Classification of acute pancreatitis—2012: revision of the Atlanta Classification and Definitions by International Consensus. Gut 2013;62:102–11.

discharged usually within the first week. Mortality is rare, and pancreatic imaging is often not required.

Moderately Severe Acute Pancreatitis

Moderately severe acute pancreatitis is defined as acute pancreatitis with transient organ failure, local complications, and/or systemic complications, but not associated with persistent (>48 hours) organ failure. The morbidity (longer stay and need for intervention) is increased; mortality is also increased somewhat (<8%) compared with that of mild acute pancreatitis, but not to the extent seen in severe acute pancreatitis. Depending on the complications of the acute pancreatitis, patients may be discharged within the second or third week or may require prolonged hospitalization because of the local or systemic complications. Noteworthy, however, is that the mortality is considerably less than that of severe acute pancreatitis.[16]

Severe Acute Pancreatitis

Severe acute pancreatitis is defined as acute pancreatitis complicated by persistent organ failure, whether the organ failure occurs in the early or late phase of the disease. Patients with severe acute pancreatitis also usually have one or more local and/or systemic complications. Of note, patients with severe acute pancreatitis that develops within the early phase (first week) are at a 36% to 50% risk of death.[9,10,17] Development of infected necrosis later in the course of the disease in patients with severe acute pancreatitis also has an extremely high mortality.[8,18]

Other groups have suggested a 2-tier or 4-tier classification of severity,[8,19,20] singling out infected necrosis as a marker of extreme severity. This system, unfortunately, overlooks a very high-risk subset of patients who have persistent organ failure within the first few days of the disease but lack any infection.

DEFINITION OF PANCREATIC AND PERIPANCREATIC COLLECTIONS

One of the biggest problems with the literature and the dialogue of acute pancreatitis is the multitude of terms used to describe the pancreatic and peripancreatic areas on cross-sectional imaging. In this classification, a crucial and important distinction is emphasized between "collections" consisting of fluid alone versus those "collections" that arise from necrosis of pancreatic parenchyma and/or peripancreatic tissues that consist of a solid component and as the necrotic process evolves, varying the degrees of fluid (**Box 2**).

Acute Peripancreatic Fluid Collection

This type of fluid collection develops in the early phase of interstitial edematous acute pancreatitis. On CECT, acute peripancreatic fluid collections (APFCs) lack a well-defined wall and are confined by the normal fascial planes in the retroperitoneum (**Fig. 5**). These fluid collections are not associated with necrotizing pancreatitis, remain sterile, and usually resolve without intervention.[21,22] When an APFC persists past 4 weeks, it is likely to develop into a pancreatic pseudocyst (see later discussion), although such development of a pseudocyst is a rare event in acute pancreatitis.

Pancreatic Pseudocyst

This term refers very specifically to a peripancreatic or, less commonly, intrapancreatic fluid collection or collections surrounded by a well-defined wall, and contains essentially no solid material (**Fig. 6**). The term pancreatic pseudocyst is very specific, and has been misused repeatedly throughout the literature and in daily dialogue. The

Box 2
Revised definitions used in this new classification

Interstitial edematous pancreatitis: Inflammation of pancreatic parenchyma and peripancreatic tissue, but without obvious tissue necrosis.

CECT Criteria

- Enhancement of the pancreatic parenchyma by contrast agent
- No evidence of peripancreatic necrosis (see below)

Necrotizing pancreatitis: Inflammation with pancreatic parenchymal necrosis and/or peripancreatic necrosis.

CECT Criteria

- Areas of pancreatic parenchymal lacking by intravenous contrast agent and/or
- Findings of peripancreatic necrosis (see below—ANC and WON)

APFC (acute peripancreatic fluid collection): Peripancreatic fluid with interstitial edematous pancreatitis and no peripancreatic necrosis. This term applies to peripancreatic fluid seen within the first 4 weeks after onset of interstitial edematous pancreatitis.

CECT Criteria

- Homogeneous collection with fluid density adjacent to pancreas confined by normal peripancreatic fascial planes
- No recognizable wall encapsulating the collection
- Occurs only in interstitial edematous pancreatitis

Pancreatic pseudocyst: Encapsulated fluid collection with minimal or no necrosis with a well-defined inflammatory wall usually outside the pancreas. This entity occurs more than 4 weeks after onset of interstitial edematous pancreatitis.

CECT Criteria

- Round or oval well circumscribed, homogeneous fluid collection
- No nonliquid component
- Well-defined wall
- Occurs after interstitial edematous pancreatitis

ANC (acute necrotic collection): A collection of both fluid and necrosis associated with necrotizing pancreatitis involving the pancreatic parenchyma and/or the peripancreatic tissues

CECT Criteria

- Heterogeneous, nonliquid density of varying degrees
- No definable encapsulating wall
- Location: intrapancreatic and/or extrapancreatic
- Occurs in setting of acute necrotizing pancreatitis

WON (walled-off necrosis): A mature, encapsulated collection of pancreatic and/or peripancreatic necrosis with a well-defined inflammatory wall occurring more than 4 weeks after onset of necrotizing pancreatitis.

CECT Criteria

- Heterogeneous liquid and nonliquid density with varying degrees of loculations
- Well-defined encapsulating wall
- Location: intrapancreatic and/or extrapancreatic
- Occurs only in setting of necrotizing pancreatitis

Modified from Banks PA, Bollen TL, Dervenis C, et al. Classification of acute pancreatitis—2012: revision of the Atlanta Classification and Definitions by International Consensus. Gut 2013;62:102–11.

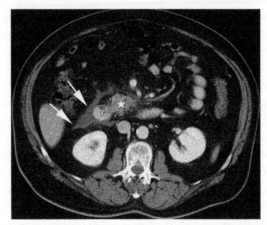

Fig. 5. A 63-year-old man with acute interstitial edematous pancreatitis and acute peri-pancreatic fluid collection (APFC) in the right anterior pararenal space (*white arrows*). The pancreatic head enhances normally (*white star*). APFC has fluid density without an encapsulating wall. D, descending part of the duodenum.

presumed etiopathogenesis of pancreatic pseudocyst is related to a disruption of the main pancreatic duct or its intrapancreatic branches without any pancreatic or peri-pancreatic necrosis evident on cross-sectional imaging. It must be stressed that development of a pancreatic pseudocyst is extremely rare in acute pancreatitis. The absence of solid material within a presumed pancreatic pseudocyst may require MRI or ultrasonography to support this diagnosis.

A special situation that can lead to a pancreatic pseudocyst in patients with necro-tizing pancreatitis involves the "disconnected duct syndrome."[23] This true fluid

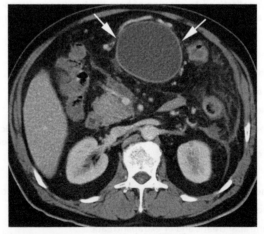

Fig. 6. A 39-year-old man with a pseudocyst 5 weeks after an episode of acute interstitial pancreatitis. Note the round, low-attenuated, homogeneous fluid collection with a well-defined enhancing rim (*white arrows* pointing at the borders of the pseudocyst) in the infe-rior recess of the lesser sac. There is absence of areas of greater attenuation, indicating nonliquid components.

collection can occur in patients when necrosis of the neck/proximal body of the pancreas isolates a still viable distal pancreatic remnant. A true pancreatic pseudocyst may develop many weeks after operative necrosectomy secondary to localized leakage of the disconnected duct into the necrosectomy cavity.

Acute Necrotic Collection

These collections occur within the first 4 weeks of the disease and contain variable amounts of fluid and solid (necrotic) material related to pancreatic and/or peripancreatic necrosis (see **Fig. 3; Fig. 7**). On CECT, acute necrotic collections (ANCs) can closely resemble an APFC in the first few days of the acute pancreatitis, but as the necrosis evolves, both fluid and solid components become evident. MRI or ultrasonography may be useful to image the solid component. An ANC is not an APFC, because it arises in patients with necrotizing pancreatitis. ANCs can be multiple, and may involve the pancreatic parenchyma alone, the peripancreatic tissue alone, or, most commonly, both the pancreatic parenchyma and the peripancreatic tissues. An ANC may be infected or sterile, and may be associated with disruption of the pancreatic ductal system with leakage of pancreatic juice into the collection, but this type of ANC is not a pancreatic pseudocyst, because an ANC contains solid material.

Walled-Off Necrosis

This type of collection consists of varying amounts of liquid and solid material surrounded by a mature, enhancing wall of reactive tissue (**Fig. 8**). A walled-off necrosis (WON) represents the mature encapsulated ANC that develops usually at least 4 weeks after onset of necrotizing acute pancreatitis. Previous terms used intermittently and inconsistently to describe this type of collection include organized pancreatic necrosis, necroma, pancreatic sequestrum, pancreatic pseudocyst with necrosis, and subacute pancreatic necrosis. Use of the term WON gathers all these terms into a common, consistent terminology.

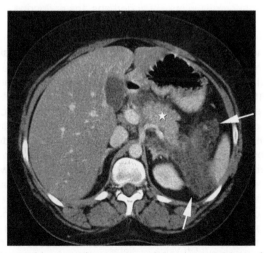

Fig. 7. ANC in a 44-year-old man with acute necrotizing pancreatitis involving only the peripancreatic tissues. The pancreatic parenchyma (*white star*) enhances normally, surrounded by a heterogeneous collection containing liquid and nonliquid components in the left retroperitoneum (*white arrows* pointing at the borders of the ANC). The ANC is not yet fully encapsulated.

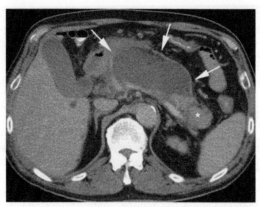

Fig. 8. A 51-year-old man with walled-off necrosis (WON) after an acute attack of acute necrotizing pancreatitis (*white star* shows normal enhancement of the pancreatic tail). A heterogeneous, fully encapsulated collection is noted in the pancreatic and peripancreatic area (*white arrows* pointing at the borders of the WON).

WON may be multiple and present at sites distant from the pancreas, and may or may not become infected. Demonstration of the presence or absence of a pancreatic ductal communication is not necessary in this classification but is of potential clinical import, because any ductal communication may affect management.

Sterile Versus Infected Necrosis

An ANC or WON can remain sterile or become infected (infected necrosis). Infection can be suspected by the clinical course of the patient (fever, leukocytosis, tachycardia) or by the presence of extraluminal gas within the areas of necrosis evident on CECT (see **Fig. 4**).

SUMMARY

The aim of this study was to update the original 1991 Atlanta Classification of acute pancreatitis to standardize the reporting and terminology of the disease and its complications. Although not necessarily commissioned by any one society, the concept of revising the prior 1991 classification received support in principle from the American Pancreatic Society, International Association of Pancreatology, European Pancreatic Club, pancreas section of the American Gastroenterological Association, Society for Surgery of the Alimentary Tract, the Pancreas Club, and several other international societies and associations interested in pancreatic disorders.

Important features of this classification have incorporated the new insights into the disease learned over the last 20 years, including the recognition that acute pancreatitis and its complications involve a dynamic process involving two phases, early and late. The accurate and consistent description of the two types of acute pancreatitis (interstitial edematous pancreatitis and necrotizing pancreatitis), its severity, and, possibly most importantly, the description of local complications based on characteristics of fluid and necrosis involving the peripancreatic collections, will help to improve the stratification and reporting of new methods of care of acute pancreatitis across different practices, geographic areas, and countries. By using a common terminology, the advancement of the science of acute pancreatitis should be facilitated.

REFERENCES

1. Bradley EL III. A clinically based classification system for acute pancreatitis. Summary of the International Symposium on Acute Pancreatitis, Atlanta, GA, September 11 through 13, 1992. Arch Surg 1993;128(5):586–90.
2. Bollen TL, van Santvoort HC, Besselink MG, et al. The Atlanta classification of acute pancreatitis revisited. Br J Surg 2008;95(1):6–21.
3. Banks PA, Bollen TL, Dervenis C, et al. Classification of acute pancreatitis—2012: revision of the Atlanta Classification and Definitions by International Consensus. Gut 2013;62:102–11.
4. Sakorafas GH, Tsiotos GG, Sarr MG. Extrapancreatic necrotizing pancreatitis with viable pancreas: a previously under-appreciated entity. J Am Coll Surg 1999; 188(6):643–8.
5. Bakker OJ, van Santvoort HC, Besselink MG, et al. Extrapancreatic necrosis without pancreatic parenchymal necrosis: a separate entity in necrotizing pancreatitis? Gut 2012. [Epub ahead of print].
6. Besselink MG, van Santvoort HC, Boermeester MA, et al. Timing and impact of infections in acute pancreatitis. Br J Surg 2009;96(3):267–73.
7. van Santvoort HC, Besselink MG, Bakker OJ, et al. A step-up approach or open necrosectomy for necrotizing pancreatitis (PANTER trial). N Engl J Med 2010;362: 1491–502.
8. Petrov MS, Shanbhag S, Chakraborty M, et al. Organ failure and infection of pancreatic necrosis as determinants of mortality in patients with acute pancreatitis. Gastroenterology 2010;139(3):813–20.
9. Johnson CD, Abu-Hilal M. Persistent organ failure during the first week as a marker of fatal outcome in acute pancreatitis. Gut 2004;53(9):1340–4.
10. Mofidi R, Duff MD, Wigmore SJ, et al. Association between early systemic inflammatory response, severity of multiorgan dysfunction and death in acute pancreatitis. Br J Surg 2006;93(6):738–44.
11. Marshall JC, Cook DJ, Christou NV, et al. Multiple organ dysfunction score: a reliable descriptor of a complex clinical outcome. Crit Care Med 1995;23(10): 1638–52.
12. Working Party of the British Society of Gastroenterology, Association of Surgeons of Great Britain and Ireland, Pancreatic Society of Great Britain and Ireland, et al. UK guidelines for the management of acute pancreatitis. Gut 2005;54(Suppl 3):iii1–9.
13. Vincent JL, Moreno R, Takala J, et al. The SOFA (Sepsis-related Organ Failure Assessment) score to describe organ dysfunction/failure. On behalf of the Working Group on Sepsis-Related Problems of the European Society of Intensive Care Medicine. Intensive Care Med 1996;22(7):707–10.
14. Muckart DJ, Bhagwanjee S. American College of Chest Physicians/Society of Critical Care Medicine Consensus Conference definitions of the systemic inflammatory response syndrome and allied disorders in relation to critically injured patients. Crit Care Med 1997;25(11):1789–95.
15. Cobb JP, O'Keefe GE. Injury research in the genomic era. Lancet 2004;363: 2076–83.
16. Vege SS, Gardner TB, Chari ST, et al. Low mortality and high morbidity in severe acute pancreatitis without organ failure: a case for revising the Atlanta classification to include "moderately severe acute pancreatitis". Am J Gastroenterol 2009; 104(3):710–5.
17. Buter A, Imrie CW, Carter CR, et al. Dynamic nature of early organ dysfunction determines outcome in acute pancreatitis. Br J Surg 2002;89(3):298–302.

18. van Santvoort HC, Bakker OJ, Bollen TL, et al. A conservative and minimally invasive approach to necrotizing pancreatitis improves outcome. Gastroenterology 2011;141:1254–63.
19. Petrov MS, Windsor JA. Classification of the severity of acute pancreatitis: how many categories make sense? Am J Gastroenterol 2010;105(1):74–6.
20. Dellinger EP, Forsmark CE, Layer P, et al, Pancreatitis Across Nations Clinical Research and Education Alliance (PANCREA). Determinant-based classification of acute pancreatitis severity: an international multidisciplinary consultation. Ann Surg 2012;256(6):875–80.
21. Balthazar EJ, Robinson DL, Megibow AJ, et al. Acute pancreatitis: value of CT in establishing prognosis. Radiology 1990;174:331–6.
22. Lenhart DK, Balthazar EJ. MDCT of acute mild (nonnecrotizing pancreatitis): abdominal complications and fate of fluid collections. Am J Roentgenol 2008; 190:643–9.
23. Pelaez-Luna M, Vege SS, Petersen BT, et al. Disconnected pancreatic duct syndrome in severe acute pancreatitis: clinical and imaging characteristics and outcomes in a cohort of 31 cases. Gastrointest Endosc 2008;68(1):91–7.

Endoscopic Management of Acute Pancreatitis

Michael H. Bahr, MD[a], Brian R. Davis, MD[b], Gary C. Vitale, MD[a],*

KEYWORDS

- Pancreatic pseudocyst • Walled-off pancreatic necrosis • Endoscopic ultrasound
- Endoscopy • Management • Acute pancreatitis

KEY POINTS

- Endoscopic direct pancreatic necrosectomy has become an essential tool in the step-up approach to treatment of acute necrotizing pancreatitis.
- Step-up approach results demonstrated a lower frequency of multisystem organ failure, major complications, and death compared with the open necrosectomy approach.
- Effective use of endoscopic therapy for treatment of acute pancreatitis eventually depends on determining optimal timing of transmural access to necrotic collections and perfecting the tools to assist in safe pancreatic debridement.

Patients presenting with acute pancreatitis can be complex on a multitude of different levels. Associated mortality rates can be 5% to 10% or more in these patients because of sepsis and multiorgan system failure.[1] Having a multifaceted approach to these patients is often necessary with radiographic, endoscopic, and surgical modalities all working to benefit the patient. Major surgical intervention can often be avoided or augmented by therapeutic and diagnostic endoscopic maneuvers. Endoscopic intervention, however, can be a double-edged sword because there is an associated risk of procedure-related acute pancreatitis. Although the quantity of information relating to the management of patients with acute pancreatitis is substantial, the data for the therapeutic role of endoscopy in patients with acute pancreatitis, in contrast to therapy for chronic pancreatitis, is less.

The diagnostic role of endoscopy in patients presenting with acute idiopathic pancreatitis can help define specific causative factors and ameliorate symptoms by endoscopic maneuvers. Etiologies of an acute pancreatitis episode, such as choledocholithiasis with or without concomitant cholangitis, microlithiasis or biliary sludge, and anatomic anomalies, such as pancreas divisum (PD) and pancreatobiliary ductal anomalies (anomalous pancreatobiliary duct junction [APBDJ], periampullary

[a] Department of Surgery, University of Louisville School of Medicine, Louisville, KY 40292, USA;
[b] Texas Tech University Health Sciences Center at El Paso, 4800 Alberta Avenue, El Paso, TX 79905, USA
* Corresponding author.
E-mail address: garyvitale@gmail.com

Surg Clin N Am 93 (2013) 563–584
http://dx.doi.org/10.1016/j.suc.2013.02.009
0039-6109/13/$ – see front matter © 2013 Elsevier Inc. All rights reserved.
surgical.theclinics.com

diverticulae, ampullary tumors, and choledochoceles), often improve after endoscopic therapy. Many of these anatomic anomalies are difficult to diagnose without endoscopic techniques, and concomitant or isolated physiologic abnormalities, such as sphincter of Oddi dysfunction, can often be diagnosed and treated endoscopically.

CAUSATIVE FACTORS OF ACUTE PANCREATITIS AND ENDOSCOPIC THERAPY

Despite a multitude of diagnostic and therapeutic advances, acute pancreatitis continues to affect more than 200,000 patients per year.[2] Most of these patients never come to procedural intervention and can be managed expectantly.[3] It has been determined that patients younger than 40 years of age having a mild first episode of pancreatitis can be followed without endoscopic intervention.[3] Should these patients have multiple episodes, or if they are older than 40 years, or have a very severe first attack then further evaluation may be considered. The severity of the initial pancreatitis episode is important to evaluate, and there are several different scoring systems to aid in objectifying a patient's severity (Ranson criteria, APACHE II, Balthazar, BISAP, Glasgow, and so forth). Severe acute pancreatitis is estimated to occur in up to 20% of patients and it is associated with sterile or infected necrosis, sepsis, and eventually progressive organ failure with a mortality rate approaching 15%.

The most common causes of acute pancreatitis especially in the Western hemisphere are related to alcohol intake and choledocholithiasis, microlithiasis, or biliary sludge. Other less common causes can be physiologic or environmental factors: hyperlipidemia with hypertriglyceridemia, drug-induced pancreatitis, autoimmune pancreatitis, and hypercalcemia. Much of these aforementioned causes, in addition to such genetic abnormalities as CFTR, PRSS1, and SPINK1 gene mutations, are discussed elsewhere in the literature. In addition, certain congenital anomalies of pancreatobiliary anatomy can contribute to recurrent episodes of acute pancreatitis, such as PD, annular pancreas, anomalous pancreatobiliary junction, and periampullary tumors.

Although much progress has been made in identifying causative factors contributing to acute pancreatitis, approximately 5% to 10% of patients still present with an undefined cause after careful evaluation.[4] The percentage of idiopathic pancreatitis has continued to decline from almost 40% historically, now down to 5% in some studies.[5] This can most likely be attributable to advances in the knowledge base, such as genetic sequencing; technologic advances, such as improved noninvasive radiographic imaging; and alternate techniques to evaluate the pancreatobiliary junction, such as endoscopic ultrasound (EUS).[1] The management of idiopathic pancreatitis can often be complex because more invasive diagnostic modalities can sometimes contribute to the very pancreatic inflammation one is trying to treat. Less invasive evaluation with magnetic resonance imaging (MRI) and EUS have certainly improved the diagnostic capabilities of modern day pancreatologists.

ENDOSCOPIC MANAGEMENT OF ACUTE BILIARY PANCREATITIS

The most common causes of acute pancreatitis in Western countries can be attributed to alcohol abuse and gallstone disease. Acute biliary pancreatitis can be exhibited in approximately 45% to 50% of patients presenting with pancreatitis.[6] Diagnosing gallstone pancreatitis can be made on serologic, radiographic, and clinical parameters. It has been shown that a patient presenting with an elevated alanine aminotransferase that is measured greater than three times the upper limit of laboratory normal approximately 1 to 2 days after the onset of symptoms is a strong predictor of biliary pancreatitis.[7] This can also be substantiated by elevated pancreatic amylase and lipase levels; typical pain patterns in these patients; and computed tomography (CT) and MRI exhibiting biliary ductal dilation, periampullary inflammation, and choledocholithiasis with or without concomitant cholelithiasis. The severity of pancreatitis is usually based on admission criteria, with no true gold standard. The modified Glasgow criteria, Ranson criteria, APACHE II scores, among other scoring systems help to differentiate those suspected of having either mild or severe disease.

THE ROLE OF URGENT ENDOSCOPIC RETROGRADE CHOLANGIOPANCREATOGRAPHY IN THE SETTING OF ACUTE BILIARY PANCREATITIS

After acute biliary pancreatitis has been proved or suggested on a clinical basis, the issue then becomes the appropriate management of this patient. Because these stones pass spontaneously soon after admission to the hospital in up to 70% of patients, the importance of early endoscopic or surgical exploration and removal of this obstructive cause has been examined in multiple randomized, controlled trials. One of the initial evaluations from Neoptolemos and colleagues[8] in 1988 examined 121 patients with acute pancreatitis thought to be caused by gallstones documented by ultrasound. These patients were randomized to either early endoscopic retrograde cholangiopancreatography (ERCP) with endoscopic sphincterotomy within the first 72 hours of admission or to conservative treatments. Although there was no significant difference in overall mortality rates between the experimental and control groups, there were significant reductions in complications (7% vs 19%) and length of hospital stay (9.5 vs 17 days) in the treatment group in this landmark study. It should be noted that gallstones were confirmed in 50 of 59 patients in the experimental group, and in 53 of 62 in the control group. Fourteen patients in the control group ultimately underwent ERCP between 6 and 30 days later, but none were done in the first 72 hours. Of these 14 patients, 3 were confirmed to have choledocholithiasis at the time of ERCP.

The results of Neoptolemos' group were subsequently re-evaluated by Fan and colleagues[9] in 1993. In this prospective, randomized trial, 195 patients underwent either urgent ERCP with sphincterotomy within 24 hours of admission (97 patients) or initially conservative treatment (98 patients). In patients in whom stones were discovered and endoscopically treated, there were fewer overall complications compared with the control group (16% vs 33%). Additionally, there was an overall reduction in mortality rate observed in the treatment group (5% vs 9%). The studies by Fan and Neoptolemos failed to exhibit a true difference in the rate of complications seen in patients with mild pancreatitis treated with early ERCP versus conservative treatment. Nowak and colleagues[10] then examined this cohort of patients and demonstrated a benefit of early ERCP in severe and mild pancreatitis. The overall complication rate (17% vs 36%) and mortality (2% vs 13%) was reduced in the treatment group. This was the first study to exhibit a clear difference between the treatment group and the control group with respect to mild and severe pancreatitis rather than just the patients with severe disease.

In contrast to the aforementioned three randomized, controlled trials that were from a single institution, the German study group with Fölsch and colleagues[11] evaluated early ERCP with sphincterotomy defined as within 72 hours of onset of symptoms versus conservative treatment across a 22-institution multicenter trial. Moreover, this multicenter study excluded patients who had either jaundice or cholangitis in contrast to the previously published reports. A total of 126 of 238 patients were randomized to the treatment group, and 112 were assigned to the control group. Early ERCP was successful in 121 of the 126, and 58 patients were found to have stones that were successfully extracted. Twenty-two of the 112 patients in the control group were ultimately treated with ERCP because of concern for choledocholithiasis, and 13 of these patients were found to have stones. The overall rate of complications was found to be similar between the two groups, but the patients in the treatment group had a higher incidence of respiratory failure and severe complications. This was the first study to dispute the use of early ERCP in patients presenting with acute biliary pancreatitis in the absence of obstructive jaundice. This study has been criticized for 19 of the 22 centers contributing less than two patients to the study, and flaws in the design and randomization process contributing to the results that differed from prior studies.

Oría and colleagues[12] again examined early endoscopic intervention compared with conservative management in patients with acute biliary pancreatitis and obstructive jaundice in one of the most recent randomized, controlled trials. Of 238 patients admitted within 48 hours after the onset of acute biliary pancreatitis, 103 were found to have biliary ductal dilation (≥ 8 mm) and obstructive jaundice (total serum bilirubin ≥ 1.20 mg/dL). These 103 patients were then randomized to receive either ERCP with endoscopic sphincterotomy (51 patients) or conservative management. Those patients with concomitant acute cholangitis were excluded from this study. The incidence of bile duct stones in the treatment group was 72%, and 40% of the patients in the conservative management group were found to have stones at the time of elective cholecystectomy. This study failed to exhibit clear benefit of early endoscopic intervention in patients with purported acute biliary pancreatitis caused by stone obstruction in the absence of acute cholangitis. There were no significant differences observed with regard to mean organ failure scores, CT severity index, incidence of local complications, and overall morbidity and mortality. Early endoscopic intervention can be detrimental, especially if the pancreatitis is unsure to be caused by stone disease or if the stone has already passed. Acute pancreatitis can often alter periampullary anatomy making ductal cannulation more difficult and can potentially contribute to a worsening of the pancreatic inflammation, increase the risk of retroperitoneal perforation, or lead to hemorrhage.

Given the results of these studies, most clinicians currently agree that patients presenting with acute biliary pancreatitis with concomitant cholangitis or suspected impacted bile duct stones benefit from early ERCP and sphincterotomy. The definition of early ERCP certainly differs, but most agree that within the first 72 hours is sufficient. The complexity arises in the preprocedural predictability of pancreatitis caused by stone disease. There is little dispute as to the benefit of early ERCP in patients with elevated liver function tests and obstructive jaundice with a septic-appearing picture and severe disease graded by an accepted scoring system, especially in those patients that have not had a cholecystectomy.

ENDOSCOPIC EVALUATION AND MANAGEMENT OF INTRINSIC ANATOMIC ABNORMALITIES CONTRIBUTING TO PANCREATITIS

Endoscopic cannulation, ultrasound, and helical CT or MRI can often reveal intrinsic anatomic abnormalities that can contribute to episodes of recurrent acute pancreatitis and eventual chronic pancreatitis. Such anomalies as PD, type 3 choledochal cysts (choledochoceles), and APBDJ all have a role in potentially leading to symptomatic acute pancreatitis that may benefit from endoscopic management.

PANCREAS DIVISUM

PD is the most commonly encountered ductal anomaly involving the pancreas. PD and other anomalies involving a dominant dorsal pancreatic duct require a keen knowledge of embryology and pancreatobiliary development. PD is defined as the lack of union of the ventral and dorsal pancreatic ducts seen in the primitive foregut of all infants. It has been estimated to occur in approximately 5% to 10% of the Caucasian population,[13] but it can be found in any race. Additionally, because of the complex migration of the ventral pancreatic bud around the primitive embryologic foregut, several variants of dorsal duct anatomy can occur.

Of the population that possesses PD, only 5% or less are symptomatic because of this ductal anomaly.[13] It is hypothesized that pancreatitis caused by PD stems from ductal hypertension and inadequate secretory drainage by the minor papilla. Although this theory of ductal hypertension makes sense and applies in the realm of other causes of acute pancreatitis, direct evidence to support this theory still remains vague and determination of which patients with PD progress to clinical symptoms is certainly multifactorial with genetic and environmental factors contributing. Moreover, the clinical picture can often be confusing because, although the signs and symptoms of chronic abdominal pain experienced by these patients seem to be pathognomonic for pancreatitis, they often do not have enzyme elevation or radiographic changes characteristic of parenchymal inflammation, so-called minimal change disease.

The clinical presentation of patients with PD varies from vague abdominal complaints to recurrent episodes of acute pancreatitis. Most of these patients are female and in the fourth decade of life.[14] The most common complaint on presentation is pain, often in the subxiphoid region with radiation around the right or left upper quadrants and to the back. This pain may or may not be associated with elevations of the patient's serum amylase, lipase, leukocyte count, or C-reactive protein. The group of patients with PD that present with chronic abdominal pain without clinically objective evidence of pancreatitis can be difficult to treat.

The diagnosis of PD can sometimes present as a challenge. Helical CT can rarely identify PD unless there is actual ductal dilation. MRI with magnetic resonance cholangiopancreatography (MRCP), with or without secretin stimulation, has a higher yield at identifying PD with a diagnostic accuracy estimated to be approximately 73%.[15] EUS and the "cross sign" seen on sonography can also aid in the diagnosis.[16] However, if the clinical suspicion is great enough, ERCP with pancreatogram still remains the most sensitive, albeit invasive method to identify PD. The diagnosis by ERCP is often confirmed by a 1- to 4-cm ventral duct that is quite diminutive in size with prominent side-branching that is often finely tapered and draining a portion of the pancreatic head and uncinate process, as would be expected from the embryologic remnant of the ventral pancreatic bud (**Fig. 1**). Cannulation of the dorsal pancreatic duct through the minor papilla is essential in the diagnosis of PD, exhibiting the typical appearance of dominant ductal drainage by the minor papilla.

After PD has been identified, the severity of symptoms and resultant pancreatitis must be assessed clinically. Like other causes of pancreatitis, patients with PD can be managed expectantly if their symptoms are mild. The sheer aspect of possessing separate dorsal and ventral pancreatic ducts does not dictate the need for intervention. The patients that have more severe episodes, exhibit clear and reproducible chronicity of symptoms, have an elevation of the pancreatic enzymes at the time of symptoms, or have a dilated dorsal duct on imaging studies may benefit from endoscopic management.

Endoscopic evaluation of PD takes a stepwise approach that often truly helps some patients long-term, whereas others have more of a diminishing return with each endoscopic intervention. There are data to suggest that those patients who possess evidence of outflow obstruction seen on ductal imaging by EUS or MRI before and after intravenous bolus of secretin may benefit from accessory sphincterotomy or

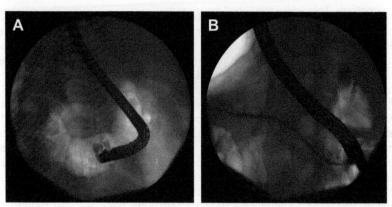

Fig. 1. Pancretograms in pancreas divisum. (A) Ventral duct pancreatogram by way of major papilla. (B) Dorsal duct pancreatogram by way of minor papilla.

operative sphincteroplasty.[17,18] Outflow obstruction from stenosis of the minor papilla is defined by persistent dilation greater than 3 mm of the dorsal pancreatic duct above the patient's baseline 10 minutes after secretin injection by MRCP in patients younger than 60 years.[17]

Endoscopic therapy for patients with PD is quite challenging. The small minor papillary orifice is often difficult to identify and cannulate. In experienced hands, cannulation of the minor papilla in patients with PD is achievable in approximately 95% of cases.[19–26] Once cannulated, there are many minor papillary manipulations that can occur: sphincterotomy, papillary dilation, stent placement, or a combination of these techniques. Isolated pneumatic balloon dilation of the minor papillary orifice without concomitant sphincterotomy or dorsal ductal stent placement has been largely abandoned because of subsequent traumatic pancreatitis.

It is the authors' practice to begin with minor papillary endoscopic sphincterotomy, with or without balloon dilation of the minor papillary orifice and stent placement. Often the ductal anatomy dictates a smaller-caliber stent be placed (5F or 7F catheter). At subsequent stent exchanges (usually done at 8-week intervals), the dorsal duct is balloon dilated and the stent is up-sized to a larger-caliber, 10F catheter stent. We continue to vary the stent lengths to minimize ductal stricture formation. If clinical symptoms improve or resolve, then the stents are removed at follow-up endoscopy. If the patient's symptoms fail to resolve after 8 weeks with a 10F catheter minor papillary stent and the duct demonstrates good contrast drainage at the time of endoscopic pancreatography, then continued endoscopic therapy is largely abandoned for alternate therapies, such as thoracoscopic splanchnicectomy or operative parenchymal resection based on their observed symptoms. We have also examined the result of endoscopic stent placement in 32 patients with symptomatic pancreatitis caused by PD during a 12-year period. Twenty-four patients were followed for approximately 60 months with a decline in pain scores, number of hospital admissions, pain medication usage, and improvement in associated symptoms, such as nausea and vomiting, observed in this study group.[13]

Minor papillary stent placement may not be entirely necessary. Stent placement may cause or exacerbate the degree of pancreatitis and complications, such as stent migration, stent occlusion, and ductal stricture with downstream pancreatic ductal dilation may result in nonresolution of symptoms. There is clear evidence to suggest that the use of minor papilla sphincterotomy alone has a favorable response in patients with acute pancreatitis caused by PD.[19–26] At a follow-up of 22 to 44 months, fewer attacks of pancreatitis and hospitalizations were shown in 76% to 94% of patients after endoscopic intervention with sphincterotomy alone.[27] Moreover, the type of sphincterotomy done (standard pull technique sphincterotomy vs a needle knife) has not exhibited any difference in treatment outcomes in a retrospective review.[27]

Early series published in the 1990s reported approximately a 20% recurrence rate of stenosis of the minor papilla after endoscopic sphincterotomy alone.[17] Multiple other studies have been performed subsequent to this to address the issue of maintaining sphincter patency with most contemporary series reporting the use of endoscopic sphincterotomy with concomitant pancreatic dorsal duct stent placement for up to approximately 18 months.[27] A retrospective evaluation comparing patients undergoing sphincterotomy alone with those undergoing sphincterotomy with dorsal duct stenting was performed. Stents were exchanged at 4-month intervals and sizes varied according to the anatomy encountered.[23] There were more treatment-related complications in the group that underwent sphincterotomy and stent placement but both groups had a decrease in the degree of chronic abdominal pain. Stenosis occurred in four patients with sphincterotomy alone and in three patients with concurrent stent placement calling into question the use of endoscopic therapy. Although this evaluation of 24 patients was small and likely underpowered, most endoscopists still consider placement of a stent into the dorsal duct as an integral part of the management of chronic abdominal pain caused by PD.

Although the focus of this article is more on endoscopic management, it is the authors' observation that those patients that benefit from ductal stenting will most likely also do well with surgical sphincteroplasty. If symptoms are relieved with stent placement, there may be a role for early transduodenal sphincteroplasty or lateral pancreaticojejunostomy if pain recurs. Many patients receive some degree of relief after dorsal duct stenting but endoscopic intervention ultimately becomes ineffective. It is the authors' observation that patients with continued pain that is not relieved after resolution of pancreatic ductal hypertension by endoscopic stenting often possess parenchymal and ductal side-branch changes more consistent with chronic pancreatitis. In these patients the authors tend to proceed with partial, if not complete, pancreatic parenchymal resection with a pancreaticoduodenectomy; subtotal pancreatectomy with pancreaticojejunostomy to drain the remaining head of the pancreas in a retrograde fashion (Duvall modification); or total pancreatectomy with or without auto-islet cell transplantation.

ANOMALOUS PANCREATICOBILIARY DUCT JUNCTION AND CHOLEDOCHOCELES

Choledochal cysts are believed to result in part from anomalies involving the junction of the biliary and pancreatic ducts. An APBDJ is usually defined as a long common channel. The pancreatic duct enters the common bile duct between 1 and 1.5 cm proximal to where the common bile duct reaches the ampulla of Vater in patients with APBDJ.[28] Greater than 90% of patients with choledochal cysts have demonstrated anomalous ductal junctions.[29,30] It is believed that the long common channel of APBDJ contributes to the reflux of pancreatic exocrine secretion into the common bile duct, and these pancreatic enzymes can be activated in the alkaline environment of the biliary system thereby resulting in degradation of the ductal mucosa and weakening of the wall of the bile duct.[30] This focal weakening can then lead to cystic degeneration of the biliary system, with multiple permutations possible. However, patients with choledochal cysts can have a normal pancreatic ductal anatomy and therefore this theory of reflux and mucosal breakdown does not always apply. It is also believed that embryologic causes contribute to the formation of these cysts because of alterations during organogenesis.

Choledochal cysts present at any age, and most are diagnosed incidentally with radiographic imaging for another purpose. The presenting symptom of these cysts often does depend on age, with obstructive jaundice being the most prominent symptom in children and abdominal pain seen in adults.[30] The Todani[31] and Alonso-Lej[32] classifications of choledochal cysts from I to V is fairly well known. Surgical resection is the mainstay in treatment of patients with extrahepatic biliary cysts because of the potential of malignant degeneration to cholangiocarcinoma observed in this population. The role of endoscopy in these patients is limited to diagnostic purposes. Therapeutic endoscopic maneuvers are limited to those patients with recurrent acute pancreatitis caused by type 3 choledochal cysts (choledochoceles), with or without an APBDJ.

Endoscopic diagnosis of a type 3 choledochal cyst can be difficult. Distinguishing between a true choledochal cyst compared with just mechanical dilation of the bile duct caused by other extrinsic factors is the main diagnostic hurdle. There have been certain criteria that had been established for the diagnosis of a type 3 choledochal cyst outlined by Park and colleagues[33]: a radiolucent halo and bulbous end to the distal common bile duct of and dynamic sequential morphologic changes with cannulation. The patients that meet at least two of these criteria are believed to have a choledochocele by fluoroscopy. There are other endoscopic findings on duodenoscopy that are suggestive of a choledochal cyst: a cystic protrusion or bulging of the duodenal lumen that has a soft, ballotable overlying mucosa and is seen to visibly enlarged during contrast infusion with cannulation is nearly pathognomonic (**Fig. 2**). It is often difficult to distinguish between choledochoceles and congenital duodenal duplication cysts unless the mucosal lining is examined histologically, but duplication cysts tend to not alter their morphology with injection of the biliary system after cannulation.

Treatment of most choledochal cysts is largely surgical. Resection, irrespective of the age of the patient, is the preferred modality of treatment. This not only obviates the need for long-term surveillance for potential malignant degeneration, but also aids in improved biliary ductal drainage and often thwarts the long-term sequelae of ductal stone disease or recurrent acute pancreatitis. However, rather than surgical resection, endoscopic management is the method of choice for patients with uncomplicated type 3 choledochal cysts (see **Fig. 2**). Patients with type 3 choledochal cysts, with or without a concomitant APBDJ (usually seen in ~90%), often benefit from just endoscopic sphincterotomy alone.[30] Choledochal cysts do carry a risk of potential malignant degeneration up to 30% even if resected, but the risk associated with choledochoceles is minimal. It has been theorized that in patients with APBDJ the enzymatic activation of exocrine secretion of the pancreatic duct by the alkaline environment of the common bile duct predisposes to altered pancreatic ductal drainage, stricture formation, calcification and potential stone formation, and pancreatic ductal hypertension. This in turn contributes to recurrent episodes of pancreatitis that are often ameliorated with endoscopic sphincterotomy.

PERIAMPULLARY DIVERTICULAE

Morphologic abnormalities at the ampulla of Vater may contribute to recurrent episodes of acute pancreatitis because of impaired drainage of exocrine secretions from the pancreatic duct. These patients present like any other case of relapsing

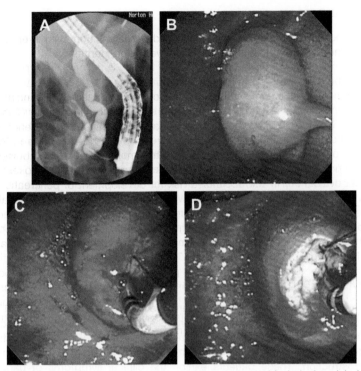

Fig. 2. Endoscopic management of a type 3 choledochal cyst (choledochocele). (*A*) Initial fluoroscopic view. (*B*) Initial endoscopic view. (*C, D*) Endoscopic sphincterotomy and opening of the cyst.

acute idiopathic pancreatitis. Radiographic evaluations with CT and MRI with MRCP can occasionally exhibit periampullary abnormalities, but diverticulae and ampullary tumors are often only diagnosed by endoscopic techniques, namely EUS and ERCP.

Periampullary diverticulae are out-pouchings of the duodenal mucosa that are located within 2 to 3 cm of the ampulla of Vater.[34] There are varying data regarding the causative factors of these diverticulae contributing to recurrent pancreatitis, but most experts agree that alterations in the duodenal mucosa around the ampulla contribute to impaired ductal drainage. After a diverticulum has been diagnosed and believed to be symptomatic, endoscopic manipulation may be attempted but is often unsuccessful because of the inability to cannulate the ducts secondary to periampullary morphologic changes. If the ampullary orifice is able to be cannulated, then such treatments as endoscopic sphincterotomy offer symptomatic relief to some patients by improving ductal drainage. The efficacy of endoscopic sphincterotomy in the treatment of patients with acute pancreatitis caused by a periampullary diverticulum was examined in a retrospective cohort of patients from Greece.[34] A total of 344 patients who had undergone ERCP between 1994 and 2005 for investigation of acute pancreatitis were retrospectively evaluated and 11 were found to have acute relapsing pancreatitis associated with a diverticulum. All of these patients underwent endoscopic sphincterotomy and were subsequently followed for recurrent attacks of pancreatitis. No further episodes were reported in all 11 patients.

AMPULLARY TUMORS

Like periampullary diverticulae, ampullary tumors can also contribute to recurrent pancreatitis and are best diagnosed endoscopically. These tumors are often found incidentally on esophagogastroduodenoscopy for reasons other than pancreatitis, and initially biopsies are taken. When dysplasia or malignancy is identified, endoscopic treatment can be useful if the tumor is small. EUS and high-resolution CT imaging can sometimes provide aid in assessing the depth of the tumor and potential resectability. Most tumors less than 3 cm, without ductal invasion, and no signs of locally advanced or distant metastatic disease can be resected en bloc endoscopically. Those patients with larger tumors, multiple tumors (eg, in patients with familial polyposis syndromes), and those with a deeper level of involvement should be referred for surgical evaluation. In the absence of ductal invasion, snare polypectomy with sphincterotomy is successful in the removal of ampullary tumors in up to 90% of cases.[28,35] Procedure-related pancreatitis has been reported in up to 30% of cases, but can be reduced by prophylactic stent placement. Although surveillance schedules differ between experts, all agree that these patients do need continued surveillance with random endoscopic biopsies.

SPHINCTER OF ODDI DYSFUNCTION AND ACUTE PANCREATITIS

Many of the aforementioned causes of recurrent acute pancreatitis are caused by mechanical or anatomic perturbations of the ampulla or pancreatic ductal orifice contributing to impaired drainage of exocrine secretions. Sphincter of Oddi dysfunction is a nonmalignant condition resulting in impairment in sphincteric physiology, leading to outflow obstruction. These patients exhibit the clinical symptoms of pancreatitis with abdominal pain, radiation, nausea, and vomiting. There is often serologic evidence of pancreatitis with elevated amylase and lipase levels, serum liver function tests, C-reactive protein, and erythrocyte sedimentation rate. These findings are frequently in the setting of a radiographically benign pancreatic parenchyma without dilated ductal anatomy and an absence of cholelithiasis. The diagnosis of Sphincter of Oddi dysfunction is confirmed by endoscopic sphincter of Oddi manometry. Selective pancreatic duct manometric pressures greater than 40 mm Hg have been found in 15% to 72% of patients with idiopathic pancreatitis.[36] Once recognized, the treatment is simply selective endoscopic sphincterotomy of the pancreatic ductal orifice, which leads to clinical improvement in up to 70% of patients.[37]

ENDOSCOPIC TREATMENT OF COMPLICATIONS OF ACUTE PANCREATITIS

Endoscopic techniques have supplanted surgery in treatment approaches for complications of acute pancreatitis including the disrupted pancreatic duct syndrome, pancreatic pseudocysts, and pancreatic necrosis. Low complication and mortality rates and the high success rate of endoscopic drainage make this approach preferable to surgery. EUS approaches decrease risks associated with endoscopic drainage of pseudocysts and facilitate the safety of endoscopic necrosectomy.

ENDOSCOPIC TREATMENT OF THE DISRUPTED DUCT SYNDROME AND FISTULAS

Disrupted pancreatic duct syndrome occurs in attacks of acute pancreatitis leading to pancreatic duct injury or from chronic pancreatitis with upstream blowout of obstructing strictures or stones.[38] Manifestations include pancreatic ascites; internal fistulae (pseudocysts, pleural effusion); or external cutaneous fistulae.[39,40] The disrupted duct syndrome demonstrates an abrupt cutoff of the pancreatic duct in patients with suspected pancreatic fistula and viable tissue visualized upstream on cross-sectional imaging. Treatment of the disrupted duct necessitates bridging of the pancreatic leak with transpapillary stents or diverting pancreatic duct flow.[41]

Endoscopic transpapillary stent bridging of duct disruption has proved effective therapy. Varadarajulu and coworkers[42] demonstrated fistula resolution of 56% with multivariate analysis showing that partial duct disruption and a bridging stent were associated with successful outcomes. Complete disruption of the pancreatic duct has less effective results with stenting as reported by Lawrence and colleagues[43] with a 59% failure of initial response or fistulae recurrence in patients with necrotizing pancreatitis. Complete duct disruptions are refractory to transpapillary stenting because the upstream disconnected segment maintains secretion without effective drainage into the duodenum.[44] Transmural drainage has arisen as the procedure of choice for complete duct disruptions that result in pseudocyst formation and fistulas to the pleura or cutaneous surface. EUS has also demonstrated effective transgastric drainage of the disconnected duct in upstream pancreatic segments resulting in pseudocysts and fistulae.[45] Further evolution of transmural EUS-assisted pancreatic duct drainage will facilitate improved outcomes in the endoscopic treatment and resolution of the disrupted duct syndrome.

PANCREATIC PSEUDOCYST DRAINAGE

Pseudocysts result from pancreatic duct disruption in up to 10% to 25% of acute pancreatitis and 20% to 40% of chronic pancreatitis cases.[46] Classification consists of fluid collections more than 4 weeks old surrounded by a nonepithelial wall of fibrous or granulation tissue (Atlanta International Symposium on Acute Pancreatitis 1993).[47] Evaluation should involve high-quality CT scan and a complete pancreatogram. Warshaw and coworkers[48] reported on experience with cystic neoplasms noting that 37% of lesions had been misdiagnosed as pseudocysts before operation. CT and MRI may help identify dependent debris suggesting pseudocyst or rim calcification indicative of neoplasm. External microlobulated morphology and internal septae were also more common in cystic neoplasms.[49] Chalian and coworkers[50] found that CT attenuation was significantly higher in pseudocysts than in mucinous neoplasms. EUS with fine-needle aspiration allows for tissue sampling and cyst fluid analysis to differentiate pseudocysts from neoplasm.[51] Vander Waaij and coworkers[52] determined in meta-analysis that carcinoembryonic antigen less than 5 ng/mL showed specificity of 95% for pseudocyst and serous cystadenoma as did carbohydrate-associated antigen Ca 19-9 concentrations of less than 37 U/mL with a specificity of 98%. Amylase was also found to be a specific predictor with a level of less than 250 U/L essentially excluding the diagnosis of pseudocyst.[53]

Indications for drainage include initial observations of Bradley and coworkers[54] that complications occurred in up to 41% of patients during an observation period of 7 weeks with spontaneous cyst resolution occurring in only 20%. Recent studies suggest that periods of prolonged observation in asymptomatic patients are safe with spontaneous resolution in up to 86% with a 3% to 9% rate of serious complications.[55,56] Data regarding pseudocyst size and outcomes are mixed, although a smaller size (<4 cm) is an important predictor of spontaneous resolution.[57] Nguyen and coworkers[58] and Cheruvu and coworkers[59] found that cyst size was not a predictor of surgical intervention resulting in recommendations that therapeutic decisions be based on symptoms of persistent pain, obstruction, ascites, pleural effusion, enlarging size, signs of infection, bleeding, or evidence of pancreatic neoplasia.

Endoscopic drainage should be considered the first preference for treatment of mature pseudocysts (**Fig. 3**). Endoscopic transpapillary drainage is beneficial for pseudocysts that communicate with the pancreatic duct, which occurs in up to 44% of pancreatograms studied by Nealon and coworkers[60,61] and when cyst size is relatively small (<6 cm). Endoscopic transmural drainage should be considered for larger cysts that fail to communicate with the duct and show signs of multiloculation and necrosis. Conventional transmural drainage can be safely performed when there is (1) evidence of gastric bulge or luminal impression, (2) absence of collateral

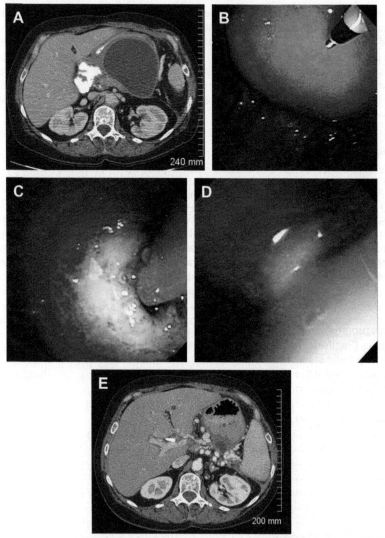

Fig. 3. Endoscopic transgastric pancreatic pseudocyst drainage. (*A*) Initial diagnostic CT with significant indentation into the stomach by the retrogastric pancreatic pseudocyst. (*B*) Endoscopic view of pseudocyst bulging into posterior gastric wall and cystotome. (*C*) Creation of cystgastrostomy and placement of wire-guided stent introducer. (*D*) Pseudocyst effluent. (*E*) Interval CT 3 months after endoscopic drainage.

blood vessels and varices, and (3) the distance from the pseudocyst to the gastric/duodenal lumen on imaging studies is less than 1 cm.[62] When pseudocysts fail to meet such criteria EUS-guided drainage has been shown to be equally successful without increased risk of complications according to Kahaleh and coworkers.[63] Recent studies by Baron and coworkers[64] have demonstrated that pseudocyst drainage is associated with higher rates of failure in infected pseudocysts and in the presence of pancreatic necrosis.

TRANSPAPILLARY DRAINAGE

Transpapillary drainage involves initial duct decompression by sphincterotomy, first on the biliary sphincter and then selectively on the pancreatic sphincter. Ancillary interventions include minor papilla sphincterotomy and dilation of duct strictures. If the pseudocyst is demonstrated on contrast injection, transpapillary endoscopic drainage is possible with placement of a large-bore (7F catheter) stent across duct disruption or within the lumen of the pseudocyst.[65] If the tail of the pancreas is visualized beyond the origin of the pseudocyst, drainage of this portion of the duct may allow pseudocyst resolution by passing a stent as far into the tail as possible beyond the connection to the pseudocyst. Transpapillary stents are left until the pseudocyst resolves or significantly decreases in size by CT scan; stents should be removed and treatment options reviewed after 6 to 8 weeks.[65] The advantage of the transpapillary approach is that the risk of gastric wall hemorrhage and retrogastric perforation is eliminated.[60]

TRANSMURAL DRAINAGE

Transmural endoscopic drainage is best indicated when pseudocysts indent the gastric or duodenal wall. Endoscopic needle localization confirms the appropriate location for cyst-enterostomy using two techniques described as a diathermic puncture and Seldinger technique.[66,67] Diathermic puncture involves either inserting a needle knife or a Cremer Cystotome (Cook Endoscopy, Winston-Salem, NC) into the gut lumen at a 90-degree angle at the maximal endoscopic bulge. A needle knife can be used to open into a bulge in the stomach (2 or 3 mm); a gush of cyst fluid is encountered when the cyst is entered; and a guidewire is then passed into the cyst cavity. A sphincterotome is passed over the wire to enlarge the opening to a minimum of 1 cm. If the mucosa is prone to bleeding with the initial cut using the needle knife, a balloon can be used to dilate the opening.[66] The Cremer Cystotome allows needle knife cyst entry followed by cyst-enterostomy creation with an electrocautery ring, and stent deployment using a single catheter.[68] The Seldinger technique involves cyst puncture by an 18-gauge needle followed by wire passage into the pseudocyst, balloon tract dilation, and stent placement. The Seldinger technique has demonstrated comparable efficacy and fewer bleeding complications compared with diathermic puncture.[67]

After completion of the cyst-enterostomy one to two 10F catheter double pigtail stents are deployed into the pseudocyst. The pigtail stents prevent migration into the cyst or out into the gastrointestinal tract. Two stents are preferable, because they allow the cyst to drain alongside the stents and through them. Transmural stents generally remain in the cavity for up to 1 year, and then they are then removed after the cyst is entirely resolved for at least 3 months by CT. If there is a small persistent pseudocyst that remains unchanged over time, the stents can also usually be removed without high risk of recurrence. Often these small cysts become isolated from the stent and the pancreatic duct. If there is a tail of the pancreas duct identified by MRI, and it is not connected to the main pancreatic duct, then one should leave the transgastric stent to drain the tail for a more prolonged period depending on the CT and ERCP anatomic findings.[69] Eventually the stent can be removed with expectation that a chronic fistula from the tail to the stomach will remain patent. It is the authors' practice to continue to evaluate patients with transpapillary, transgastric, or transduodenal stents placed for pancreatic pseudocysts with a CT scan periodically. After the cyst has resolved by imaging and the patient's symptoms have improved or resolved, then the stents are removed endoscopically. If the symptoms do not improve or if there is no diminution in the size of the cyst after at least 6 months, then surgical intervention is considered.

Pseudocysts that do not present with a lumenal bulge or that present with perigastric varices are best drained under direct ultrasound guidance. EUS is used for direct needle-guided puncture of the pseudocyst with a 19-gauge needle followed by wire placement, dilation over the guidewire, and stent placement. Kahaleh and coworkers[63] demonstrated 93% effective drainage with EUS in patients lacking a lumenal bulge or presenting with portal hypertension. A novel device for single-step cyst-enterostomy has been developed (Navix; Xlumena, San Francisco, CA), which permits needle puncture followed by entry of an anchoring and dilating balloon to allow double wire advancement for sequential stent placement.[70]

Endoscopic drainage of pancreatic fluid collections has been demonstrated as effective in large retrospective patient series. Hookey and coworkers[71] described results in 116 patients demonstrating equivalent efficacy between transmural and transpapillary drainage techniques. Antillon and coworkers[72] demonstrated successful 82% single-step EUS-guided transmural endoscopic drainage of simple and complex pancreatic pseudocysts. Weckman and coworkers[73] demonstrated an 86% rate of successful pseudocyst drainage in 165 patients with a 5% recurrence rate during a 25-month follow-up. Cahen and coworkers[69] noted that independent predictors of successful outcomes included location of the cyst in the pancreatic head, insertion of multiple stents into the pseudocyst cavity, and stent drainage of the pseudocyst cavity longer than 6 weeks. Predictors of failure included the presence of moderate abscess debris. Large numbers of series have demonstrated that endoscopic drainage is successful with between 71% and 95% complete pseudocyst resolution, complications between 0% and 37%, and 0% and 1% procedure-related mortality.[60,62,63,69,71–73]

Pancreatic abscesses can also be effectively treated with endoscopic drainage. According to the Atlanta classification pancreatic abscesses are circumscribed intra-abdominal collections of pus containing little or no pancreatic necrosis.[47] Necrotic residual debris has been described as the most important factor in predicting failure of endoscopic drainage.[63] Endoscopic abscess drainage was initially reported by Binmoeller and coworkers[60] demonstrating an 80% complete resolution rate. Vitale and coworkers[74] demonstrate an initial success rate of 94% for drainage of pancreatic abscesses followed by an overall success rate of 80% on long-term follow-up; there was a 20% recurrence that required surgery. Weckman and colleagues[73] noted similar efficacy between endoscopic pseudocyst and abscess drainage except that abscesses required multiple stents and repeated endoscopic drainage procedures. Baron (2002) described treatment of pancreatic fluid collections with necrotic debris defined as walled-off pancreatic necrosis (WOPN) with lower success rates of 71% and higher recurrence rates of 29%.[64] Effective measures to facilitate drainage of necrotic debris include placement of large-bore covered self-expanding metallic stents and nasocystic tubes for irrigation debridement.[68]

On long-term follow-up, endoscopic drainage has a reported recurrence rate ranging from 8% to 20%, which compares favorably with recurrence rates reported after surgical cyst-enterostomy (5%–20%).[62,63,69,75–78] After a 44-month follow-up,

Sharma and colleagues[75] reported the results of endoscopic drainage for 38 pseudo-cysts. Three patients had symptomatic recurrences, whereas three had asymptomatic recurrences; all had alcohol-induced pancreatitis. No recurrences were seen in the biliary pancreatitis and trauma group. With a median follow-up of 26 months, De Palma and coworkers[76] showed a 20.9% of recurrence rate. Causes of recurrent pseudocysts usually involve the obstruction of a cystoenterostomy or stent obstruc-tion in the presence of persistent pancreatic disease or ductal stricture.

Complications of endoscopic pseudocyst drainage include retroperitoneal perfora-tion, bleeding, and infection. Sharma and colleagues[75] report experience in 38 pa-tients with endoscopic drainage. Massive bleeding in one patient required surgery, whereas stent blockage and pseudocyst infection in three patients and perforation in one patient were managed conservatively. De Palma and coworkers[76] also report an experience with 49 patients using an endoscopic approach. Twelve (24.5%) pa-tients had complications: two patients had bleeding, two patients had mild pancrea-titis, and eight patients had cyst infections. Five patients with infection had pancreatic necrosis and three patients had a clogged stent. In our experience, a wide opening of the cyst enterostomy (about 1–2 cm) is necessary in potentially infected cases to reduce the incidence of infected cyst complications.[74]

ENDOSCOPIC NECROSECTOMY

Endoscopic access to pancreatic fluid collections has had limited efficacy in the pres-ence of significant pancreatic necrosis leading to classifications of WOPN and tech-niques of endoscopic direct pancreatic necrosectomy.[63] The New Atlanta Classification of pancreatic fluid collections divides into acute phase (first 4 weeks) and chronic phase.[77] Chronic collections are divided into pseudocysts and WOPN, which comprise heterogeneous collections of necrotic debris and an encapsulating wall. Indications for endoscopic drainage of pancreatic fluid collections most impor-tantly include suspected infection in patients with systemic clinical deterioration and multiple organ failure.[79] Interventions within the first few weeks of necrotizing pancre-atitis generally have poor outcomes with a guiding principle to delay endoscopic pancreatic debridement until fluid collections have become encapsulated.[80] A recently published multicenter series demonstrated a 95% successful resolution rate for endoscopic necrosectomy for WOPN with a median duration between initial pancreatitis to endoscopic intervention of 46 days. Direct correlation was demon-strated between successful endoscopic therapy and the degree of encapsulation of WOPN.[81]

The advent of transmural endoscopic therapy for pancreatic necrosis began with the use of linear echoendoscopes. Siefert and coworkers[82] reported the first cases of direct endoscopic necrosectomy with endoscopic cavitary debridement. Papach-ristou and coworkers[83] described early treatment of pancreatic necrosis for 53 pa-tients with necrotic pancreatic fluid collections an average of 49 days after the onset of necrotizing pancreatitis with an 81% success rate. The largest series to date presents from six American centers with a resolution rate in WOPN of 91% with a mean number of 3.7 procedures with 2.5 debridements.[81] This multicenter study demonstrated complications of pneumoperitoneum (13%) and bleeding (18%). Other reported complications include infection (undrained necrosis); pancrea-titis; aspiration; stent migration; occlusion; pancreatic duct damage; and complica-tions of sedation.[80] Overall complication rates for direct endoscopic drainage or direct pancreatic necrosectomy have been reported as between 15% and 25% for experienced practitioners.[84]

Direct endoscopic necrosectomy uses multiple endoscopic tools to achieve adequate debridement usually resulting in serial procedures as pancreatic necrosis liquefies and patients experience worsening organ failure (**Fig. 4**).[85] Transmural access can be obtained using standard access techniques or under EUS guidance. EUS guidance is recommended in cases involving extensive necrotic debris for

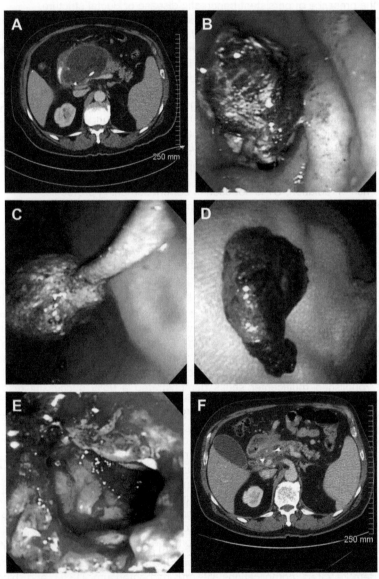

Fig. 4. Endoscopic transduodenal pancreatic necrosectomy. (*A*) Interval CT scan after initial ERCP with attempted transpapillary drainage. (*B*) Endoscopic view of pancreatic necrosum into first portion of duodenum. (*C*) Debridement and retrieval of pancreatic necrosum with Roth net. (*D*) Extracorporeal specimen of pancreatic necrosum. (*E*) Final endoscopic view of necrotic cavity after debridement. (*F*) Completion CT 3 months after necrosectomy.

adequate identification of mural blood vessels. Evidence suggests that EUS allows for higher efficacy and fewer complications for nonbulging collections, collections in the tail, and in patients with varices.[62] The site for transmural access should be through a wall less than 10 mm in thickness. After the collection is accessed the enterostomy can be dilated with low-profile controlled radial expanding balloons, biliary dilating catheters, or a Soehendra stent extractor. The goal of dilation is to achieve a fistula tract of 20 mm diameter at the time of initial drainage.[85]

Completion of the cyst-enterostomy or fistula is followed by fluid aspiration for Gram stain and culture to direct antibiotic therapy. A forward-viewing gastroscope can then be driven across the gastric or duodenal wall to perform direct necrosectomy. Necrotic pancreas can then be removed using snares, baskets, and water-jets. Hydrogen peroxide can also be used for irrigation to liquefy the debris.[84] Devitalized tissue is debrided serially removing as much tissue as safely possible at each session with deposition in the stomach or duodenum. Stents are left after each procedure to mature the fistula tract to allow debridement by gastric and bile acids. Uncovered metal stents have been used for fistula tract maturation. Recent case series from Japan have introduced a novel uncovered metallic stent for serial access to pancreatic pseudocysts and WOPN. This metallic stent allows serial access for necrosectomy and has a low profile, which prevents complications of stent migration and erosion.[86]

Endoscopic direct pancreatic necrosectomy has become an essential tool in the step-up approach to treatment of acute necrotizing pancreatitis. The Dutch Acute Pancreatitis Study Group initially demonstrated the efficacy of the step-up approach where patients with pancreatic necrosis were randomized to open necrosectomy compared with minimally invasive retroperitoneal drainage therapies. Step-up approach results demonstrated a lower frequency of multisystem organ failure, major complications, and death compared with the open necrosectomy approach.[87] The Dutch group subsequently published the PENGUIN trial that randomized patients to endoscopic transgastric versus open necrosectomy. This study demonstrated improved outcomes in the endoscopic necrosectomy group with lower incidence of major complications to include new-onset multiple organ failure, intra-abdominal bleeding, enterocutaneous fistula or pancreatic fistulas, or death when compared with the surgical group.[88] Effective use of endoscopic therapy for treatment of acute pancreatitis will eventually depend on determining optimal timing of transmural access to necrotic collections and perfecting the tools to assist in safe pancreatic debridement.

REFERENCES

1. Kozarek RA. Role of ERCP in acute pancreatitis. Gastrointest Endosc 2002;56(6): S231–6.
2. Fagenholz PJ, Castillo CF, Harris NS, et al. Increasing United States hospital admissions for acute pancreatitis, 1988-2003. Ann Epidemiol 2007;17:491–7.
3. Ballinger AB, Barnes E, Alstead EM, et al. Is intervention necessary after a first episode of acute idiopathic pancreatitis? Gut 1996;38:293–5.
4. Draganov P, Forsmark CE. Idiopathic pancreatitis. Gastroenterology 2005;128(3): 756–63.
5. Baillie J. What should be done with idiopathic recurrent pancreatitis that remains "idiopathic" after standard investigation? JOP 2001;2:401–5.
6. Lankisch PG, Schirren CA, Schmidt H, et al. Etiology and incidence of acute pancreatitis: a 20-year study in a single institution. Digestion 1989;44:20–5.

7. Tenner S, Dubner H, Steinberg W. Predicting gallstone pancreatitis with labora-tory parameters: a metaanalysis. Am J Gastroenterol 1994;89(10):1863–6.

8. Neoptolemos JP, London NJ, James D, et al. Controlled trial of urgent ERCP and endoscopic sphincterotomy versus conservative treatment for acute pancreatitis due to gallstones. Lancet 1988;2:979–83.

9. Fan ST, Lai EC, Mok FP, et al. Early treatment of acute biliary pancreatitis by endo-scopic papillotomy. N Engl J Med 1993;328:228–32.

10. Nowak A, Nowakowska-Dulawa E, Marek T, et al. Final results of the prospec-tive, randomzed, controlled study on endoscopic sphincterotomy versus conven-tional management in acute biliary pancreatitis. Gastroenterology 1995;108: A380.

11. Fölsch UR, Nitsche R, Ludtke R, et al. Early ERCP and papillotomy compared with conservative treatment for acute biliary pancreatitis. N Engl J Med 1997; 336:237–42.

12. Oría A, Cimmino D, Ocampo C, et al. Early endoscopic intervention versus early conservative management in patients with acute gallstone pancreatitis and bilio-pancreatic obstruction: a randomized trial. Ann Surg 2007;245(1):10–7.

13. Vitale GC, Vitale M, Vitale DS, et al. Long-tern follow-up of endoscopic stenting in patients with chronic pancreatitis secondary to pancreas divisum. Surg Endosc 2007;21:2199–202.

14. Howard TJ. Pancreas divisum and other variants of dominant dorsal duct anat-omy. In: Cameron JL, Cameron AM, editors. Current surgery therapy. 10th edition. Philadelphia: Elsevier Saunders; 2011. p. 393–8.

15. Matos C, Meten T, Devière J, et al. Pancreas divisum: evaluation with secretin-enhanced magnetic resonance cholangiopancreatography. Gastrointest Endosc 2001;53:728–33.

16. Rana SS, Gonen C, Villmann P. Endoscopic ultrasound and pancreas divisum. JOP 2012;13(3):252–7.

17. Warshaw AL, Simeone JF, Schapiro RH, et al. Evaluation and treatment of the domi-nant dorsal duct syndrome (pancreas divisum redefined). Am J Surg 1990;159: 59–66.

18. Mosler P, Fogel EL, McHenry L, et al. Accuracy of magnetic resonance cholan-giopancreatography in the diagnosis of pancreas divisum. Gastrointest Endosc 2005;61(5):AB100.

19. Coleman SD, Gisen GM, Troughton AB, et al. Endoscopic treatment of pancreas divisum. Am J Gastroenterol 1994;89:1152–5.

20. Siegel JH, Ben-Zvi JS, Pullano W, et al. Effectiveness of endoscopic drainage for pancreas divisum: endoscopic and surgical results in 31 patients. Endoscopy 1990;22:129–33.

21. Gerke H, Byrne MF, Stiffler HL, et al. Outcome of endoscopic minor papillotomy in patients with symptomatic pancreas divisum. JOP 2004;5:122–31.

22. Lehman GA, Sherman S, Nisi R, et al. Pancreas divisum: results of minor papilla sphincterotomy. Gastrointest Endosc 1992;39:1–8.

23. Heyries L, Barthet M, Delvasto C, et al. Long-term results of endoscopic manage-ment of pancreas divisum with recurrent acute pancreatitis. Gastrointest Endosc 2002;5:376–81.

24. Lans JI, Geenan JE, Johanson JF, et al. Endoscopic therapy in patients with pancreas divisum and acute pancreatitis: a prospective, randomized, controlled trial. Gastrointest Endosc 1992;38:430–4.

25. Kozarek RA, Ball TJ, Patterson DJ, et al. Endoscopic approach to pancreas divi-sum. Dig Dis Sci 1995;40:1974–81.

26. Saltzman JR. Endoscopic treatment of pancreas divisum: why, when, and how? Gastrointest Endosc 2006;64(5):712–5.
27. Fogel EL, Toth TG, Lehman GA, et al. Does endoscopic therapy favorably affect the outcome of patients who have recurrent acute pancreatitis and pancreas divisum? Pancreas 2007;34(1):21–45.
28. Attasaranya S, Abdel Aziz AM, Lehman GA. Endoscopic management of acute and chronic pancreatitis. Surg Clin North Am 2007;87:1379–402.
29. Samavedy R, Sherman S, Lehman GA. Endoscopic therapy in anomalous pancretobiliary duct junction. Gastrointest Endosc 1999;50(5):623–7.
30. Ladas SD, Katsogridakis I, Tassios T, et al. Choledochocele. An overlooked diagnosis: report of 15 cases and review of 56 published reports from 1984-1992. Endoscopy 1995;27:233–9.
31. Todani T, Watanabe Y, Narusue M, et al. Congenital bile duct cysts: classification, operative procedures and review of thirty-seven cases including cancer arising from choledochal cyst. Am J Surg 1977;134:263–9.
32. Alonso-Lej F, Rever WB, Pessagno DJ. Congenital choledochal cyst, with report of two and analysis of 94 cases. Int Abstr Surg 1959;108:1–30.
33. Park KB, Auh YH, Kim JH, et al. Diagnostic pitfall in the cholangiographic quality and its effect on visualization. Abdom Imaging 2001;26(1):48–54.
34. Katsinelos P, Paroutoglou G, Chatzimavroudis G, et al. Endoscopic sphincterotomy for acute relapsing pancreatitis associated with periampullary diverticula: a long-term follow-up. Acta Gastroenterol Belg 2007;70(2):195–8.
35. Adler DG, Baron TH, Davila RE, et al. ASGE guideline: the role of ERCP in disease of the biliary tract and the pancreas. Gastrointest Endosc 2005;62(1):1–8.
36. Behar J, Corazziari E, Guelrud M, et al. Functional gallbladder and sphincter of Oddi disorders. Gastroenterology 2006;130(5):1498–509.
37. Sgouros SN, Pereira SP. Systematic review: sphincter of Oddi dysfunction-noninvasive diagnostic methods and long-term outcome after endoscopic sphincterotomy. Aliment Pharmacol Ther 2006;24:237–46.
38. Deviere J, Busco H, Baize M, et al. Complete disruption of the main pancreatic duct: endoscopic management. Gastrointest Endosc 1995;42:445–51.
39. Bracher GA, Manocha AP, De Banto JR, et al. Endoscopic pancreatic duct stenting to treat pancreatic ascites. Gastrointest Endosc 1999;49(6):710–5.
40. Cooper ST, Malick J, McGrath K, et al. EUS-guided rendezvous for the treatment of pancreticopleural fistula in a patient with chronic pancreatitis and pancreas pseudodivisum. Gastrointest Endosc 2010;71(3):652–4.
41. Kozarek RA, Ball TJ, Patterson DJ, et al. Endoscopic transpapillary therapy for disrupted pancreatic duct and peripancreatic fluid collections. Gastroenterology 1991;100:1362–70.
42. Varadarajulu S, Noone TC, Tutuian R, et al. Predictors of outcome in pancreatic duct disruption managed by endoscopic transpapillary stent placement. Gastrointest Endosc 2005;61:568–75.
43. Lawrence C, Howell DA, Stefan AM, et al. Disconnected pancreatic tail syndrome: potential for endoscopic therapy and results of long-term follow-up. Gastrointest Endosc 2008;67:673–9.
44. Telford JJ, Farrell JJ, Saltzman JR, et al. Pancreatic stent placement for duct disruption. Gastrointest Endosc 2002;56:18–24.
45. Fabbri C, Luigiano C, Maimone A, et al. Endoscopic ultrasound-guided drainage of pancreatic fluid collections. World J Gastrointest Endosc 2012;4(11):479–88.
46. O'Malley VP, Cannon JP, Postier RG. Pancreatic pseudocysts: cause, therapy and results. Am J Surg 1985;150:680–2.

47. Bradley EL III. A clinically based classification system for acute pancreatitis. Summary of the International Symposium on Acute Pancreatitis. Arch Surg 1993;128:586–90.
48. Warshaw AL, Compton CC, Lewandrowski KB, et al. Cystic tumors of the pancreas. Ann Surg 1990;212:432–43.
49. Macari M, Finn ME, Bennett GL, et al. Differentiating pancreatic cystic neoplasms from pancreatic pseudocysts at MR imaging: value of perceived internal debris. Radiology 2009;251:77–84.
50. Chalian H, Torre HG, Miller FH, et al. CT attenuation of unilocular pancreatic cystic lesions to differentiate pseudocysts from mucin-containing cysts. JOP 2011;12: 384–8.
51. Ahmad NA, Kochman ML, Lewis JD, et al. Can EUS alone differentiate between malignant and benign cystic lesions of the pancreas? Am J Gastroenterol 2001; 96:3295–300.
52. Van der Waaij LA, van Dullerman HM, Porte RJ. Cyst fluid analysis in the differential diagnosis of pancreatic cystic lesions: a pooled analysis. Gastrointest Endosc 2005;62:383–9.
53. Brugge WR, Lewandrowski K, Lee- Lewandrowski E, et al. Diagnosis of pancreatic cystic neoplasms: a report of the cooperative pancreatic cyst study. Gastroenterology 2004;126:1330–6.
54. Bradley EL III, Clements JL Jr, Gonzalez AC. The natural history of pancreatic pseudocysts: a unified concept of management. Am J Surg 1979;137:135–41.
55. Vitas GH, Sarr MG. Selected management of pancreatic pseudocysts: operative versus expectant management. Surgery 1992;111:123–30.
56. Yeo CJ, Bastidas JA, Lynch Nyham A, et al. The natural history of pancreatic pseudocysts documented by computed tomography. Surg Gynecol Obstet 1990;170:411–7.
57. Beebe DS, Bubrick MP, Onstad GR, et al. Management of pancreatic pseudocysts. Surg Gynecol Obstet 1984;159:562–4.
58. Nguyen BL, Thompson JS, Edney JA, et al. Influence of the etiology of pancreatitis on the natural history of pancreatic pseudocysts. Am J Surg 1991;162: 527–30.
59. Cheruvu CV, Clarke MG, Prentice M, et al. Conservative treatment as an option in the management of pancreatic pseudocysts. Ann R Coll Surg Engl 2003;85:313–6.
60. Binmoeller KF, Siefert H, Walter A, et al. Transpapillary and transmural drainage of pancreatic pseudocysts. Gastrointest Endosc 1995;42:219.
61. Nealon WH, Walser E. Main pancreatic ductal anatomy can direct choice of modality for treating pancreatic pseudocysts (surgery versus percutaneous drainage). Ann Surg 2002;235:751–8.
62. Melman L, Azar R, Beddow K, et al. Primary and overall success rates for clinical outcomes after laparoscopic, endoscopic and open pancreatic cystgastrostomy for pancreatic pseudocysts. Surg Endosc 2009;23:267–71.
63. Kahaleh M, Shami VM, Conaway MR, et al. Endoscopic ultrasound drainage of pancreatic pseudocyst: a prospective comparison with conventional endoscopic drainage. Endoscopy 2006;38:355–9.
64. Baron TH, Harewood GC, Morgan DE, et al. Outcome differences after endoscopic drainage of pancreatic necrosis, acute pancreatic pseudocysts and chronic pancreatic pseudocysts. Gastrointest Endosc 2002;56:7–17.
65. Catalano MF, Geenen JE, Schmalz MJ, et al. Treatment of pancreatic pseudocysts with ductal communication by transpapillary pancreatic duct endoprosthesis. Gastrointest Endosc 1995;42:214–8.

66. Howell DA, Holbrook RF, Bosco JJ, et al. Endoscopic needle localization of pancreatic pseudocysts before transmural drainage. Gastrointest Endosc 1993;39:693–8.
67. Monkemuller KE, Baron TH, Morgan DE. Transmural drainage of pancreatic fluid collections without electrocautery using the Seldinger technique. Gastrointest Endosc 1998;48:195–200.
68. Seewald S, Ang TL, Soehendra N. Advanced techniques of drainage of peripancreatic fluid collections. Gastrointest Endosc 2009;69(Suppl 2):S182–5.
69. Cahen D, Rauws E, Fockens P, et al. Endoscopic drainage of pancreatic pseudocysts: long-term outcome and procedural factors associated with safe and successful treatment. Endoscopy 2005;35:977–83.
70. Binmoeller KF, Weilert F, Marson F, et al. EUS-guided transluminal drainage of pancreatic pseudocysts using the NAVIX access device and two plastic stents: initial clinical experience. Gastrointest Endosc 2011;73:AB331.
71. Hookey LC, Debroux S, Delhaye M, et al. Endoscopic drainage of pancreatic-fluid collections in 116 patients: a comparison of etiologies, drainage techniques and outcomes. Gastrointest Endosc 2006;63:635–43.
72. Antillon MR, Shah RJ, Stiegmann G, et al. Single-step EUS-guided transmural drainage of simple and complicated pancreatic pseudocysts. Gastrointest Endosc 2006;63:797–803.
73. Weckman L, Kylanpaa ML, Poulakkainen P, et al. Endoscopic treatment of pancreatic pseudocysts. Surg Endosc 2006;20:603–7.
74. Vitale GC, Davis BR, Vitale M, et al. Natural orifice translumenal endoscopic drainage for pancreatic abscess. Surg Endosc 2009;23:140–6.
75. Sharma SS, Bhargawa N, Govil A. Endoscopic management of pancreatic pseudocyst: a long-term follow-up. Endoscopy 2002;34:203.
76. De Palma GD, Galloro G, Puzziello A, et al. Personal experience with endoscopic treatment of pancreatic pseudocysts. Long-term results an analysis of prognostic factors. Minerva Chir 2001;56:475 [in Italian].
77. Hansen BO, Schmidt PN. New classification of acute pancreatitis. Ugeskr Laeger 2011;173:42–4.
78. Aljarabah M, Ammori BJ. Laparoscopic and endoscopic approaches for drainage of pancreatic pseudocysts: a systematic review of published series. Surg Endosc 2007;21(11):1936–44.
79. Van Santvoort HC, Baker OJ, Bollen TL, et al. A conservative and minimally invasive approach to necrotizing pancreatitis improves outcomes. Gastroenterology 2011;141:1254–63.
80. Takahashi N, Papachristou GI, Schmit GD, et al. CT findings of walled-off pancreatic necrosis (WOPN): differentiation from pseudocyst and prediction of outcome after endoscopic therapy. Eur Radiol 2008;18:2522–9.
81. Gardner TB, Coelho-Prabhu N, Gordon SR, et al. Direct endoscopic necrosectomy for the treatment of walled-off pancreatic necrosis: results from a multicenter US series. Gastrointest Endosc 2011;73:718–26.
82. Seifert H, Wehrmann T, Schmitt T, et al. Retroperitoneal endoscopic debridement for infected pancreatic necrosis. Lancet 2000;356:653–5.
83. Papachristou GI, Takahashi N, Chahal P, et al. Peroral endoscopic drainage/debridement of walled-off pancreatic necrosis. Ann Surg 2007;245:943–51.
84. Seifert H, Biermer M, Schmitt W, et al. Transluminal endoscopic necrosectomy after acute pancreatitis: a multicenter study with long-term follow-up (the GEPARD Study). Gut 2009;58:1260–6.
85. Gardner TB. Endoscopic management of necrotizing pancreatitis. Gastrointest Endosc 2012;76(6):1214–23.

86. Itoi T, Binmoeller KF, Shah J, et al. Clinical evaluation of a novel lumen-apposing metal stent for endosonography guided pancreatic pseudocyst and gallbladder drainage (with videos). Gastrointest Endosc 2012;75(4):870–6.

87. Van Santvoort HC, Besselink MG, Bakker OJ, et al. A step-up approach or open necrosectomy for necrotizing pancreatitis. N Engl J Med 2010;362:1491–502.

88. Baker OJ, van Santvoort HC, Burnschot S, et al. Endoscopic transgastric versus surgical necrostectomy for infected necrotizing pancreatitis. JAMA 2012;307: 1053–61.

The Role of Antimicrobial Therapy in Severe Acute Pancreatitis

Thomas J. Howard, MD

KEYWORDS

- Severe acute pancreatitis • Infected pancreatic necrosis • Prophylactic antibiotics
- Systemic inflammatory response syndrome • Secondary pancreatic infection
- Computed tomography-guided fine needle aspiration

KEY POINTS

- Pancreatic necrosis is prone to secondary microbial infection (infected pancreatic necrosis) with organisms found in the gastrointestinal tract (gram-negative organisms, gram-positive organisms, anaerobes, and fungi).
- Empiric broad-spectrum antimicrobial treatment of patients for clinical deterioration while awaiting final culture results is called treatment on demand.
- At this time, there is no compelling evidence that the use of prophylactic antibiotics in patients with severe acute pancreatitis is efficacious.
- Quinolones plus metronidazole or carbapenems are the initial drugs of choice to treat secondary pancreatic infections.
- Fungal organisms are found in up to 25% of cultures from infected pancreatic necrosis and are best treated with diflucan.
- When carefully applied, fine needle aspiration Gram's stain and culture are useful for diagnosing secondary pancreatic infections.

SEVERE ACUTE PANCREATITIS

Acute pancreatitis is an inflammatory disease of the pancreas caused by a variety of etiologic factors, with alcohol, gallstones, and idiopathic factors being the most common in the United States. The pancreatic inflammation incites a complex and variable host response, resulting in a disease course can be either mild and self-limiting (80%), or severe and necrotizing (20%).[1,2] In mild acute pancreatitis, patients experience the abrupt onset of abdominal pain, nausea, and vomiting, which gradually subside over a 3- to 5-day period. Treatment consist of nothing by mouth (NPO), intravenous fluid hydration, pain control, supplemental oxygenation, and antiemetics to manage symptoms while the pancreatic inflammation subsides and the gland returns to normal structure and function. Antimicrobials play no role in this disease process.[1] In contrast,

Hepatobiliary Surgical Cancer Care, Community Hospital North, 8040 Clearvista Parkway, Suite 240, Indianapolis, IN 46256, USA
E-mail address: tomjohnhoward@gmail.com

Surg Clin N Am 93 (2013) 585–593
http://dx.doi.org/10.1016/j.suc.2013.02.006
0039-6109/13/$ – see front matter © 2013 Elsevier Inc. All rights reserved.
surgical.theclinics.com

severe acute pancreatitis (SAP) (**Box 1**) results in microcirculatory disturbances within the pancreatic parenchyma,[3] leading to tissue ischemia and regional cell death best quantified by contrast-enhanced computed tomography (CECT) as pancreatic and peripancreatic necrosis (**Fig. 1**).[4] Prognostic estimates on an individual patient's clinical course can be made by the volume, location, and infection status of the necrosis. While sterile pancreatic necrosis can be localized and compartmentalized by the body, infected pancreatic necrosis (IPN) serves as a nidus for bacteria and fungus, which is thought to be the key driver of organ failure, systemic sepsis, and death.[5-7]

PATHOPHYSIOLOGY OF SECONDARY PANCREATIC INFECTIONS

Loss of both pancreatic parenchyma and its associated exocrine duct system allows leakage of pancreatic enzymes into the retroperitoneum, inciting further inflammation, fat necrosis, and fluid sequestration. It is within these areas of devitalized tissue (pancreatic and peripancreatic necrosis) and fluid (postnecrotic pancreatic fluid collections) where secondary pancreatic infections with bacteria or fungus can occur[8] The at-risk population for secondary pancreatic infection includes those patients with necrosis of more than 30% of their gland based on CECT, while patients with lesser volumes of necrosis have a good chance for resolution.[4] Although the exact mechanisms contributing to secondary pancreatic infections remain uncertain, the predominant cultured pathogens imply an origin from the gastrointestinal (GI) tract.[8-10] Gastric microbial colonization combined with alterations in intestinal permeability can lead to microbial translocation, which has been hypothesized as a mechanism for secondary pancreatic infections.[11] This hypothesis, if true, might explain why both early enteral nutrition[12] and selective gut decontamination[13] have shown beneficial effects in decreasing secondary pancreatic infections in this setting.

CLINICAL COURSE OF SAP

The clinical course of patients with SAP can be divided into 2 phases.[14] There is an early cytokine-mediated phase (within the first week of onset), distinguished by frequently reversible organ failure (most commonly pulmonary and/or renal) that is a consequence of the systemic inflammatory response syndrome (SIRS).[15] In this early disease phase, deaths are attributable to MOD, mediated predominately by cytokines rather than infection.[16] Volume resuscitation, organ support, enteral nutrition, and the search for a treatable cause of MOD (eg, bacteremia, pneumonia, ischemic colitis, or

---

Box 1
Definition for SAP

- ≥30% pancreatic necrosis of CECT

    or

- Noncontrast scans with extensive or multiple peripancreatic fluid collections and pancreatic edema (Bathazar grade E)

    and either

- C-reactive protein (CRP) >120 mg/L

    or

- Multiple organ dysfunction (MOD) score >2

Data from Refs.[4,30,39]

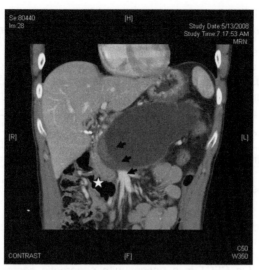

Fig. 1. CECT scan showing >70% necrosis of the pancreatic parenchyma seen as lack of contrast enhancement (*black arrows*) when compared with the perfused pancreatic parenchyma (*white star*).

gangrenous cholecystitis) are the main focus of treatment during this disease phase.[9] If antibiotics are used in this setting, they are targeted at active infection (eg, bacteremia, pneumonia, or gangrenous cholecystitis) or started empirically (on demand) for a 72-hour course in a critically ill patient who is spiking fevers or deteriorating without an obvious source of infection.[17] This use of antibiotics is common in critically ill patients in the intensive care unit and has been estimated to decrease mortality by up to 50% in patients with gram-negative sepsis. In this early time period following the onset of SAP, infected pancreatic necrosis is unusual, while infections in the lungs, kidneys/bladder, or blood stream predominate.[9] Once the source of infection is accurately identified, targeted antibiotic therapy and source control (eg, line change or cholecystectomy) can be instituted.

The second clinical phase of the disease occurs later (usually 2–4 weeks following onset), when patients develop systemic sepsis (fevers, tachycardia, or leukocytosis) combined with either persistent or new-onset MOD. Secondary pancreatic infection with bacterial and/or fungal organisms is a likely cause for this clinical deterioration.[7,9] The development of infected pancreatic necrosis has been shown to peak between weeks 2 and 4.[8] While secondary pancreatic infections (IPN and infected postnecrotic pancreatic fluid collections [IPNPFC]) are important complications in this secondary disease phase of SAP, other infectious complications can occur, requiring a thorough investigation for other possible sources of infection (blood, urine, invasive lines, or stool) (**Table 1**). If IPN is suspected, making a firm and accurate diagnosis is essential, as early intervention (<4 weeks after disease onset) in patients with pancreatic necrosis (particularly major open operations) has been associated with a poor clinical outcome.[9,14,18,19]

DIAGNOSIS OF SECONDARY PANCREATIC INFECTION

IPN requires a prompt accurate diagnosis, targeted antimicrobial therapy, and a step-up approach to therapeutic intervention.[8,18] Only a positive culture or Gram's stain

Table 1
Type of infectious complication, incidence, and timing of complications in 65 patients with SAP

Infectious Complications	Incidence of Complication	Timing of Complication After Onset of SAP
IPN	47% (31/65)	17.6 + 2.9 d
Pneumonia	28% (18/65)	10.7 + 2.5 d
Bacteremia	11% (7/65)	13.7 + 1.5 d
GI tract	8% (5/65)	16.8 + 3.9 d
Urinary tract infection	6% (4/65)	20.5 + 4.8 d

Data from Xue P, Deng LH, Zhang ZD, et al. Infectious complications in patients with severe acute pancreatitis. Dig Dis Sci 2009;54(12):2748–53.

from image-guided (CT or ultrasound) percutaneous fine-needle aspiration (FNA) or direct necrosectomy serves as definitive evidence of a secondary pancreatic infection.[20,21] Occasionally, the presence of extraluminal gas (small air bubbles) in the non-enhancing areas of a CECT in a patient with pancreatic necrosis can be highly suggestive of infection, assuming that the extraluminal air is a consequence of gas-forming organisms in the necrosis and not localized GI tract perforation. In both instances, while the necrosis is infected, in certain situations with a localized perforation, the necrosis is able to slough into the GI tract and resolve as a consequence of an unplanned internal drainage. Although FNA can be very useful in certain situations, several caveats need to be considered. The indications for, timing of, and frequency of repeated FNA in patients with SAP are topics of considerable debate.[22] Because of these uncertainties, specific guidelines for use of CT-guided FNA for early detection of infected pancreatic necrosis have not been clearly established.[14] FNA is associated with a false-negative rate of approximately 10%, and although false positives can theoretically occur, they are extremely rare. Therefore, a single negative FNA should not be relied upon to rule out secondary pancreatic infection and should be repeated if the clinical suspicion for infection remains high. Lastly, FNA carries a small but real risk of contaminating sterile necrosis with bacteria. In an appropriate setting, during a single aspiration, this risk seems acceptable; however, frequent repeated aspirations should be discouraged. Given these considerations, image-directed FNA for Gram's stain and culture should only be obtained in the situation where the result (either positive or negative) is going to directly impact treatment decisions. There are circumstances where experienced pancreatic surgeons will manage patients throughout their entire clinical course without image-directed FNA, choosing instead to follow patients clinically for resolution of symptoms and their return to wellness. In those patients who remain unwell (pain, inability to eat, organ dysfunction) despite 3 to 4 weeks of medical managment and who have large volumes of retroperitoneal debris (necrosis) benefit from necrosectomy as further medical care is unlikely to result in resolution of the patient's symptoms.

MICROBIOLOGY OF SECONDARY PANCREATIC INFECTION

The organisms most commonly cultured from secondary pancreatic infections include: gram-negative aerobic coliform bacteria (*Escherichia coli, Klebsiella, Enterobacteriacea*), gram-positive aerobic bacteria (*Staphylococcus, Streptococcus*) and fungi (*Candida* species) (**Table 2**). Anaerobic bacteria have been cultured in approximately 8% to 15% of patients, while fungal infections are present in 20% to 25% of

Table 2
Common microbiologic isolates from IPN

	Gram-Negative Bacteria	Gram-Positive Bacteria	Fungal Organisms
Aerobe	*Escherichia coli* *Klebsiella pneumonia* *Enterobacteriacea* *Proteus sp.* *Pseudomonas aureginosa* *Citrobacter sp.* *Serratia sp.*	*Enterococcus sp.* *Staphylococcus aureus* *Staphylococcus epidermidis* *Streptococcus sp.*	*Candida albicans* *Candida glabrata*
Anaerobe	*Bacteroides sp.*	*Peptostreptococcus* *Clostridia perfringens*	

Gram-negative isolates—35%–55%.
Gram-positive isolates—20%–35%.
Anaerobic isolates—8%–15%.
Fungal isolates—20%–25%.
Data from Refs.[8,19,23–26]

patients.[8,19,23–26] There is some evidence that following the introduction and routine use of prophylactic antibiotics in the 1990s, the bacteriology of secondary pancreatic infections shifted from gram-negative coliforms toward more gram-positive infections (ie, *Staphylococcus epidermidis*), resistant bacteria (ie, methicillin-resistant *Staphylococcus aureus* [MRSA], vancomycin-resistant *Enterococcus* [VRE]), and fungi.[13,23–25,27] This shift is important to note when one is selecting broad antimicrobial coverage to treat potential pathogens in an on-demand fashion before definitive culture results being available. In spite of this changing bacteriologic spectrum, there are few data to suggest that infected pancreatic necrosis with antibiotic-resistant organisms (eg, MRSA or VRE) has any worse outcome following appropriate treatment and source control than infected pancreatic necrosis with antibiotic-sensitive organisms.[23,28,29] In contrast, there are some data to suggest that secondary bacterial infection with *Candida* is associated with an increased in-hospital mortality rate.[24,27]

PROPHYLACTIC ANTIBIOTICS IN SAP

The role of antibiotic prophylaxis in SAP has undergone a cyclical evolution. Early prospective, clinical trials in the 1970s failed to show a benefit in mortality rate using prophylactic antibiotics in patients with acute pancreatitis, although these studies were justly criticized for the inclusion of patients with mild forms of pancreatitis and the use of ampicillin, a drug subsequently shown to not penetrate sufficiently into the pancreas.[30] With the development of powerful new antibiotics against enteric organisms in the 1990s, coupled with better laboratory and imaging methods to stratify the clinical severity of an episode of pancreatitis, use of prophylactic antibiotics in patients with SAP was again tried.

Support for this practice began to appear with the publication of small prospective randomized clinical trials showing that administration of prophylactic antibiotics in patients with SAP could reduce the incidence of pancreatic infections,[31] reduce both infection rates and mortality,[32] or reduce pancreatic infections, need for operation, and late mortality. These clinical trials were small, used different drugs on different schedules, measured different outcomes, and lacked appropriate placebo controls. Despite these methodological difficulties, pooling of these trials under the rubric of a meta-analysis showed a benefit for antibiotic prophylaxis.[33]

In 2004 a large, prospective multi-institutional placebo-controlled double-blind trial of 114 patients with SAP randomized to ciprofloxacin and metronidazole or placebo was published showing no benefit to antibiotic prophylaxis in preventing infection in pancreatic necrosis.[25] Following this, a second, similarly well-designed trial by Dellinger and colleagues[34] echoed these prior findings, namely, there that is no statistically significant benefit to the use of early prophylactic antibiotic in patients with SAP. One of the findings in these trials is that the equivalent outcomes between treatment and control groups in both studies spawned the idea that antibiotics given to critically ill patients on demand during the course of their hospital stay may be just as effective as continuous prophylactic antibiotics.[25] Early and extensive use of broad-spectrum prophylactic antibiotics in critically ill patients should be discouraged unless there is compelling evidence as to their benefit.[34] Currently, this level of evidence does not exist. The combined weight of these last 2 clinical trials will undoubtedly skew any future meta-analysis against routine prophylactic antibiotic use, making the current recommendations from the critical care society against routine prophylactic antibiotics especially prophetic.[35]

ANTIMICROBIAL SELECTION AND TREATMENT

The spectrum of antibiotics chosen to treat IPN should include coverage for both aerobic gram-negative and gram-positive bacteria and anaerobes (see **Table 1**). When choosing appropriate antibiotic coverage, care should be taken to consider the classes of antibiotics that have optimal penetration into pancreatic tissue. Three groups of antibiotics have been carefully studied in this regard analyzing their penetration into the human pancreas when given intravenously in both the normal and inflamed pancreas.[36] Aminoglycoside antibiotics (eg, netilmicin and tobramycin) in standard intravenous dosages fail to penetrate into the pancreas in sufficient tissue concentrations to cover the minimal inhibitory concentration (MIC) of the bacteria that are commonly found in secondary pancreatic infections. Acylureidopenicillins (mezlocillin and piperacillin) and third-generation cephalosporins (ceftizoxime and cefotaxime) have an intermediate penetration into pancreas tissue but are such effective bactericidal agents against gram-negative microorganisms that even with slightly lower tissue concentrations they can cover the MIC for most gram-negative organisms found in pancreatic infections. Unfortunately, these compounds as a group are much less effective against gram-positive bacteria and anaerobes. If used, they should optimally be paired with drugs used to treat gram-positive bacteria or anaerobes. Quinolones (ciprofloxacin and ofloxacin) and carbapenems (imipenem) both show good tissue penetration into the pancreas as well as broad-spectrum bactericidal activity against gram-negative and gram-positive bacteria. Carbapenems have the additional benefit of excellent anaerobic coverage. Metronidazole, with its bactericidal spectrum focused almost exclusively against anaerobes, also shows good penetration into the pancreas. Given these pharmacokinetic and microbial spectrum data, quinolones plus metronidazole or carbapenems should be the initial drugs of choice to treat secondary pancreatic infections.[25,34]

Prophylactic antifungal coverage should be considered in all severely ill surgical patients with multiple risk factors for invasive candidiasis due to the substantial and convincing data for its efficacy.[37] Much less clear at present is whether these recommendations for *Candida* prophylaxis in surgical patients should be broadened to include their use in severely ill patients with pancreatic necrosis.[38] Patients with yeast on Gram's stain following CT-guided FNA or direct culture at the time of necrosectomy should receive fluconazole targeted at *Candida albicans*, the most common fungal isolate in secondary pancreatic infections. *Candida glabrata,* which has a higher MIC for fluconazole than *C albicans,* should be treated either with a higher dose of fluconazole (400 mg/d) to achieve greater concentrations in the pancreas, or caspofungin. Those patients who have been treated with fluconazole prophylactically and subsequently develop infected necrosis with yeast should be treated with caspofungin.[38]

Although initiation of antimicrobial therapy may be difficult, stopping antibiotics often times proves even more challenging, as there are currently no tools available to guide antibiotic therapy.[39] The clinical criteria used to initiate antibiotic treatment in patients with a predicted severe course of acute pancreatitis include: newly developed sepsis or SIRS, newly developed failure of 2 or more organ systems, proven pancreatic or extrapancreatic infection, or an increase in serum C-reactive protein in combination with evidence of pancreatic or extrapancreatic infections.[25] The clinical criteria to stop antimicrobial therapy in surgical patients have classically been the absence of fever and a normal white blood cell count. Secondary pancreatic infection in a patient with pancreatic necrosis in the past was considered an absolute indication for open pancreatic necrosectomy.[19] Over the last decade, there has developed a more nuanced appreciation of the complex relationship between infection, the patient, and the approach and timing of intervention. Currently, in critically ill patients with early onset secondary pancreatic infection (<2 weeks), percutaneous drainage and antibiotics can be effective until the patient's clinical course can be stabilized to allow for definitive necrosectomy. Several new minimally invasive techniques are available for necrosectomy, and these can optimally be delayed until the third or fourth week after disease onset, limiting the perioperative morbidity and mortality.[39] Although there are scattered reports in the literature of patients with documented secondary pancreatic infections who have been treated successfully by antimicrobial therapy alone,[40] most clinicians believe that intervention via a step-up approach is an important adjunct to antimicrobial therapy for optimal source control.[18]

REFERENCES

1. Baron TH, Morgan DE. Acute necrotizing pancreatitis. N Engl J Med 1999; 340(18):1412–7.
2. Guzman EA, Rudnicki M. Intricacies of host response in acute pancreatitis. J Am Coll Surg 2006;202(3):509–19.
3. Klar E, Endrich B, Messmer K. Microcirculation of the pancreas. A quantitative study of physiology and changes in pancreatitis. Int J Microcirc Clin Exp 1990; 9:85–101.
4. Balthazar EJ. Acute pancreatitis: assessment of severity with clinical and CT evaluation. Radiology 2002;223:603–13.
5. Johnson CD, Abu-Hilal M. Persistent organ failure during the first week as a marker of fatal outcome in acute pancreatitis. Gut 2004;53:1340–4.
6. Lytras D, Manes K, Triantopouilou C, et al. Persistent early organ failure: defining the high-risk group of patients with severe acute pancreatitis? Pancreas 2008;36: 249–54.
7. Gloor B, Müller CA, Worni M, et al. Later mortality in patients with severe acute pancreatitis. Br J Surg 2001;88:975–9.
8. Beger HG, Bittner R, Block S, et al. Bacterial contamination of pancreatic necrosis: a prospective clinical study. Gastroenterology 1986;91:433–8.
9. Besselink MG, van Santvoort HC, Boermeester MA, et al. Timing and impact of infections in acute pancreatitis. Br J Surg 2009;96:267–73.

10. Xue P, Deng LH, Zhang ZD, et al. Infectious complications in patients with severe acute pancreatitis. Dig Dis Sci 2009;54(12):2748–53.

11. McNaught CE, Woodcock MP, Mitchell J, et al. Gastric colonization, intestinal permeability and septic morbidity in acute pancreatitis. Pancreatology 2002;2: 463–8.

12. Petrov MS, VanSantvoort HC, Besselink MG, et al. Enteral nutrition and the risk of mortality and infectious complication in patients with severe acute pancreatitisL a meta-analysis of randomized trials. Arch Surg 2008;143(11):1111–7.

13. Luiten EJ, Hop WC, Lange JF, et al. Controlled clinical trial of selective decontamination for the treatment of severe acute pancreatitis. Ann Surg 1995;222:57–65.

14. Uhl W, Warshaw A, Imrie C, et al. IAP guidelines for the surgical management of acute pancreatitis. Pancreatology 2002;2:565–73.

15. Buter A, Imrie CW, Carter CR, et al. Dynamic nature of early organ dysfunction determines outcome in acute pancreatitis. Br J Surg 2002;89:298–302.

16. Neoptolemos JP, Raraty M, Finch M, et al. Acute pancreatitis: the substantial human and financial costs. Gut 1998;42:886–91.

17. Dunn DL. Gram-negative bacterial sepsis and sepsis syndrome. Surg Clin North Am 1994;74:621–35.

18. van Santvoort HC, Besselink MG, Bakker OJ, et al. A step-up approach or open necrosectomy for necrotizing pancreatitis. N Engl J Med 2010;362:1491–502.

19. Büchler MW, Gloor B, Müller CA, et al. Acute necrotizing pancreatitis: treatment strategy according to the status of infection. Ann Surg 2000;232(5):619–26.

20. Gerzof SG, Banks PA, Robbins AH, et al. Early diagnosis of pancreatic infection by computed tomography-guided aspiration. Gastroenterology 1987;93:1315–20.

21. Rau B, Pralle U, Mayer JM, et al. Role of ultrasonographically guided fine-needle aspiration cytology in the diagnosis of infected pancreatic necrosis. Br J Surg 1998;85:179–84.

22. Pappas TN. Con: computerized tomographic aspiration of infected pancreatic necrosis: the opinion against its routine use. Am J Gastroenterol 2005;100(11): 2373–4.

23. Howard TJ, Temple MB. Prophylactic antibiotics alter the bacteriology of infected necrosis in severe acute pancreatitis. J Am Coll Surg 2002;195:759–67.

24. Isenmann R, Schwarz M, Rau B, et al. Characteristics of infection with *Candida* species in patients with necrotizing pancreatitis. World J Surg 2002;25:372–6.

25. Isenmann R, Rünzi M, Kron M, et al. Prophylactic antibiotic treatment in patients with predicted severe acute pancreatitis: a placebo-controlled, double blind trial. Gastroenterology 2004;126:997–1004.

26. Lumsden A, Bradley EL. Secondary pancreatic infections. Surg Gynecol Obstet 1990;170:459–67.

27. Hoerauf A, Hammer S, Muller-Myshok B, et al. Intra-abdominal candida infection during acute necrotizing pancreatitis has a high prevalence and is associated with increased mortality. Crit Care Med 1998;26:2010–5.

28. Gloor B, Müller CA, Worni M, et al. Pancreatic infection in severe pancreatitis: the role of fungus and multi-resistant organism. Arch Surg 2001;136:592–6.

29. DeWaele JJ. Rational use of antimicrobials in patients with severe acute pancreatitis. Semin Respir Crit Care Med 2011;32(2):174–80.

30. Bradley EL. Antibiotics in acute pancreatitis: current status and future directions. Am J Surg 1989;158:472–8.

31. Pederzoli P, Bassi C, Vesentini S, et al. A randomized multicenter clinical trial of antibiotic prophylaxis of septic complications in acute necrotizing pancreatitis with imipenem. Surg Gynecol Obstet 1993;176:480–3.

32. Sainio V, Kemppaninen E, Puolakkainen P, et al. Early antibiotic treatment in acute necrotizing pancreatitis. Lancet 1995;346:663–7.
33. Golub R, Siddiqui F, Pohl D. Role of antibiotics in acute pancreatitis: a meta-analysis. J Gastrointest Surg 1998;2:496–503.
34. Dellinger EP, Tellado JM, Soto NE, et al. Early antibiotic treatment for severe acute necrotizing pancreatitis: randomized, double-blind, placebo-controlled study. Ann Surg 2007;245:674–83.
35. Nathens AB, Curtis JR, Beal RJ, et al. Management of the critically ill patient with severe acute pancreatitis. Crit Care Med 2004;32:2524–36.
36. Büchler M, Malfertheiner P, Friess H, et al. Human pancreatic tissue concentration of bactericidal antibiotics. Gastroenterology 1992;103:1902–8.
37. Pittet D, Monod M, Suter PM, et al. *Candida* colonization and subsequent infections in critically ill surgical patients. Ann Surg 1994;220:751–8.
38. Solomkin JS, Umanskiy K. Intraabdominal sepsis: newer interventional antimicrobial therapies for infected necrotizing pancreatitis. Curr Opin Crit Care 2003;9: 424–7.
39. Besselink MG, van Santvoort HC, Witteman BJ, et al. Management of severe acute pancreatitis: it's all about timing. Curr Opin Crit Care 2007;13:200–6.
40. Adler DG, Chari ST, Dahl TJ, et al. Conservative management of infected necrosis complicating severe acute pancreatitis. Am J Gastroenterol 2003;98:98–103.

Operative Management of Acute Pancreatitis

Ronald F. Martin, MD[a,b,*], Amanda R. Hein, MD[a]

KEYWORDS

• Acute pancreatitis • Management • Necrosis • Pseudocysts • Pancreatic resection
• Pseudocyst drainage

KEY POINTS

- The operative management of acute pancreatitis is focused on managing the acute complications, the long-term sequelae, or the prevention of recurrent pancreatitis.
- Using the least amount of intervention to achieve the stated goals has always been the case; however, the evolution of videoscopic and endoscopic techniques have greatly expanded the tools available.
- Patience, vigilance, expertise, judgment, and an ability to be humbled are necessary for the successful practitioner who manages patients with severe pancreatitis.

Acute pancreatitis is more of a range of diseases than it is a single pathologic entity. Its clinical manifestations range from mild, perhaps even subclinical, symptoms to a life-threatening or life-ending process. The classification of acute pancreatitis and its forms are discussed in fuller detail by Sarr and colleagues elsewhere in this issue. For the purposes of this discussion, the focus is on the operative interventions for acute pancreatitis and its attendant disorders.

The most important thing to consider when contemplating operative management for acute pancreatitis is that we do not operate as much for the acute inflammatory process as for the complications that may arise from inflammation of the pancreas. In brief, the complications are related to: necrosis of the parenchyma, infection of the pancreas or surrounding tissue, failure of pancreatic juice to safely find its way to the lumen of the alimentary tract, erosion into vascular or other structures, and a persistent systemic inflammatory state. The operations may be divided into three major categories: those designed to ameliorate the emergent problems associated with the ongoing inflammatory state, those designed to ameliorate chronic sequelae

[a] Department of General Surgery, Marshfield Clinics and Saint Joseph's Hospital, 1000 North Oak Avenue, Marshfield, WI 54449, USA; [b] Department of Surgery, University of Wisconsin School of Medicine and Public Health, 640 Highland Avenue, Madison, WI, USA
* Corresponding author. Department of General Surgery, Marshfield Clinics and Saint Joseph's Hospital, 1000 North Oak Avenue, Marshfield, WI 54449.
E-mail address: martin.ronald@marshfieldclinic.org

Surg Clin N Am 93 (2013) 595–610
http://dx.doi.org/10.1016/j.suc.2013.02.007
0039-6109/13/$ – see front matter © 2013 Elsevier Inc. All rights reserved.
surgical.theclinics.com

of an inflammatory event, and those designed to prevent a subsequent episode of acute pancreatitis. This article provides a review of the above.

ACUTE PANCREATITIS

Acute pancreatitis may be histologically classified as either interstitial or necrotizing edematous, each of which have its unique complications.[1] Acute pancreatic inflammation will progress to pancreatic necrosis in approximately 20% to 30% of patients with severe acute pancreatitis.[2] The terminology used to describe acute pancreatitis and its consequences has a long history of being less than well standardized. Over the past 20 years or so, attempts at using standardized descriptions have been markedly improved. In another article by Sarr and colleagues in this issue, the most recent consensus agreements are reviewed in detail. Pancreatic necrosis is defined by the International Symposium on Acute Pancreatitis as the presence of one or more diffuse or focal areas of nonviable pancreatic parenchyma, usually associated with peripancreatic fat necrosis.[2] The Acute Pancreatitis Classification Working Group has further elaborated on this in defining three distinct subgroups: pancreatic parenchymal and associated peripancreatic necrosis, pancreatic parenchymal necrosis alone, or peripancreatic necrosis alone. All of these can be either sterile or infected.[2]

Walled-off necrosis, formerly referred to as organized pancreatic necrosis, is a well-circumscribed collection of purulent material in close proximity to the pancreas that develops greater than 4 weeks after an episode of necrotizing pancreatitis. It is due to secondary infection of liquefied necrosis that then becomes walled off.[3–8] It is generally a highly viscous collection and contains liquid and solid or semisolid debris.

Pancreatic ductal disruptions may develop in up to 50% of patients who have acute necrotizing pancreatitis and may lead to peripancreatic fluid collections. Loss of ductal integrity may lead to further necrosis, infection, or fistulization.[9–11] The persistent leakage of pancreatic fluid may result in pseudocyst formation (a bounded collection) or diffuse leakage into the retroperitoneum yielding worsening inflammation, leakage into the peritoneal cavity resulting in pancreatic ascites, or leakage into the thorax resulting in pancreatic pleural effusion. The latter two phenomena are essentially pathognomonic for main pancreatic ductal disruption.

Disconnected tail syndrome is defined by a complete disruption of the main pancreatic duct (demonstrated by loss of opacification of the duct or inability to place a guidewire into the distal duct) and CT imaging demonstrating contrast-enhancing viable pancreatic tissue upstream from the disruption.[9] A nonhealing pancreatic fistula, pseudocyst, or fluid collection despite a course of conservative medical management is added to the definition by some investigators.[12] The downstream pancreas can drain via the papilla or retrograde into a fluid collection or fistula, whereas the upstream pancreas will drain aberrantly until the drainage is redirected or that section of pancreas is removed or atrophies.[9] Of note: the nomenclature that is conventionally used for the pancreas and its ducts is potentially confusing. The generally accepted anatomic principal of referring to proximal and distal based on direction of flow is completely ignored when referring to the pancreas. In the opinion of the corresponding author, correcting this and renaming some operations accordingly would be optimal. However, this is most unlikely to occur.

The cause of acute pancreatitis is most often related to gallstones or ethanol use, though a myriad of other causes have been identified. In the United States, gallstone pancreatitis is the most common form of acute pancreatitis due to transient obstruction at the ampulla or from increased pancreatic ductal pressure secondary to persistent stone impaction or ampullary scarring secondary to stone passage.[13,14]

Operations and Indications

As mentioned above, the operations used for acute pancreatitis are designed to manage the complications in the acute phase, the long-term sequelae, or prevention of subsequent episodes of acute pancreatitis. In this section, procedures used in the acute phase of inflammation are discussed. These operations are mostly aimed at removing dead or devitalized tissue, removing or draining infected solid or semisolid tissue, draining pus, and/or providing a safer avenue for egress of pancreatic secretions. Although much is written about these procedures, and there always seems to be more confusion than necessary about these operations, they are really quite straightforward in nature. Some simple principles pertain: all infected material must go; the degree of containment, or lack thereof, of the suspect material must be considered; the viscosity of the problematic tissue or fluid collection influences choices; and consideration of draining or resecting potentially sterile fluid or tissue invariably is a clinical judgment based on the overall status of the patient.

PANCREATIC NECROSIS

Pancreatic necrosis results from insufficient perfusion of pancreatic parenchyma to support metabolic requirements. There are many models of how this actually happens and they are discussed by Sarr and colleagues elsewhere in this issue in greater detail. Necrosis of the pancreas may be relatively minor and self-limiting or it may progress to a more substantial and potentially life-threatening process.[15] Although pancreatic necrosis remains sterile, the main indications for intervention are an uncontrolled systemic inflammatory response syndrome (SIRS) or significant question over whether the presumption of sterility is secure. It is generally accepted that infected pancreatic necrosis is an indication for intervention.[15] Over the past several years, the enthusiasm for early operative intervention in suspected sterile necrosis has waned because, even in the setting of multiorgan failure, many studies have shown that operative management does not confer significant mortality benefit and may actually increase morbidity. The rare indications for intervention in sterile necrosis include worsening organ failure despite maximal support, inability to tolerate enteral nutrition, weight loss, worsening jaundice, fevers, or failure to improve after 4 to 6 weeks of nonoperative management.[16]

In the setting of infected, possibly infected, or worsening sterile necrosis, debridement is preferred to resection in an attempt to preserve as much functional organ as possible.[16] Also, attempts at an anatomic resection in the setting of severe acute pancreatitis are frequently not technically possible and are likely to yield more complications than they resolve. The survival rate is generally improved the longer operative management can be delayed– unless, of course, clear evidence of significant infection is present. This is likely due to better demarcation resulting in removal of less vital tissue and less bleeding. Some investigators have suggested that optimal outcomes have been realized when surgery can be delayed for at least 1 month.[14,17] The only randomized controlled trial comparing debridement within the first 72 hours with debridement after at least 12 days was terminated early; however, preliminary data demonstrated a mortality of 56% for the early group and 27% for the late group.[16] In the authors' experience, the main benefit from waiting, when possible, to operate is reducing the number of operations required to achieve the main clinical objectives.

Significant complication rates in cases associated with pancreatic debridement include: pancreatic fistula in 41% to 50%; exocrine insufficiency in 20%; endocrine insufficiency in 16%; enteric fistulas in greater than 10%; postoperative hemorrhage in 3% to 20%; prolonged postoperative hospitalization, typically greater than 1 month; and greater than 4 months before return to regular activities.[2,18,19] Surgical debridement is associated with an overall morbidity rate of 19% to 62% and a mortality rate of 6% to 28%.[2,19]

Technical Considerations in Managing Pancreatic Necrosis

The technical choices made in the management of pancreatic necrosis must always be made with some basic principles in mind. First, be mindful of the desired end state— removal of all devitalized and infected tissue in the setting of an alive patient. Second, achieve the first goal in the least invasive and least traumatic way possible. Einstein is quoted as saying, "Everything should be made as simple as possible but not simpler." The same philosophy applies to pancreatic debridement; it should be as minimally invasive as possible but not more so. If achieving the clinical objectives in a timely and cost-effective manner requires a more invasive procedural choice, then do so. Using minimally invasive techniques for the sake of doing so misses the point altogether.

Open Necrosectomy

Open approach to necrosectomy can be done in many ways. One approach includes a necrosectomy and closure with standard surgical drains that are left in place for an average of 7 days. Reoperation is performed on an as-needed basis. Reports of this technique show a mortality rate of 4% to 19%.[14] Some investigators suggest abandoning this approach because of inadequate debridement and a 40% incidence of reinfection.[14] However, other contributors feel this technique may be sufficient for very small, well-delineated processes.[15] The open or semiopen technique includes necrosectomy combined with open packing and scheduled repeat laparotomies, usually every 48 hours, until all necrotic tissue has been removed. Followed by closure, or not, of the abdomen depending on the clinical circumstances. This technique has a high reported rate of postoperative complications, including pancreatic fistulas, bowel compromise, and bleeding, as well as mortality rate of 4% to 18%.[14] The closed technique entails necrosectomy with extensive intraoperative lavage of the pancreatic bed followed by closure over large-bore drains for continued postoperative high-volume lavage of the lesser sac. Reports of this technique suggest lower mortality rates of 7% to 9% compared with other open procedures.[14]

Although all the techniques listed above can and do work, the literature reporting their relative effectiveness may be difficult to compare. Even attempts at carefully controlled studies are challenging in patients with these maladies. Also, in the corresponding author's opinion, it may be impossible to control for all the operative and surgical variation that inherently exists in the management of these patients.

Minimally Invasive Surgery Approach for Necrosis

As in all other areas of surgery, minimally invasive approaches are gaining popularity in the management of pancreatic necrosis. Potential benefits claimed are: minimizing operative trauma; decreased incidence of incisional hernias; avoidance of bacterial contamination and translocation, thereby improving the postoperative septic response; and decreasing the need for ICU care.[14,20] Some of these claims may be aspirational over actual. To date, no survival benefit over open procedures has been clearly demonstrated.[20] Potential limitations include poor surgical exposure, difficulty removing solid or highly viscous necrotic tissue through small ports, loss of tactile guidance, need for multiple procedures, longer overall hospital stays, and need for reliance on interventional radiology.[20]

The semiopen technique uses a retroperitoneal approach via a small 5 cm incision. The Dutch Acute Pancreatitis Study Group has compared this technique to open necrosectomy with continuous postoperative lavage. They found favorable outcomes in the semiopen group, which developed less postoperative multiorgan failure and demonstrated a trend toward decreased mortality. In addition, there was no difference in the number of procedures required between the two groups.[21]

Videoscopic options include transperitoneal or retroperitoneal approaches.[14] The retroperitoneal approach potentially avoids peritoneal contamination and is typically done after a period of CT-guided drainage. One major disadvantage of this approach is the inability to perform other intraabdominal procedures such as cholecystectomy or jejunostomy tube placement.[14] With the transperitoneal approach, the lesser sac is explored via a transmesocolic route.[14] At the conclusion of either of these procedures, drains are left in place for postoperative drainage and/or lavage.[14] There are no randomized controlled trials showing that the laparoscopic approach is superior to open surgery; however, the theoretical advantages include less postoperative pain, shorter length of stay, and earlier return to normal activities.[14]

Transgastric Resection or Drainage

When necrosis and/or fluid collections are contained and limited to the lesser sac they may be approached by a transgastric technique. Transgastric drainage or debridement of the lesser sac can be achieved by open, videoscopic, or endoscopic means. As with other procedures, the choice will not be just based on the tools available and the technical expertise of the operator but also, and more importantly, on the nature and viscosity of the material to be removed.

A step-up approach for controlling the liquid component (pus) of infection, instead of treating the definitive source, is sometimes used as a temporary measure en route to removing the infected necrotic tissue. The first step is to drain the collection of infected fluid using either percutaneous or endoscopic means to mitigate sepsis. If this does not lead to clinical improvement, the next step is minimally invasive retroperitoneal necrosectomy or open necrosectomy. A multicenter trial conducted in 2010 randomized 88 subjects with suspected or confirmed infected necrosis to undergo primary open necrosectomy or a step-up approach. The primary endpoints were major complication or death, which occurred in 69% of subjects assigned to open necrosectomy compared with 40% of those in the step-up group. Of subjects in the step-up approach group, 35% required only percutaneous drainage. New-onset multiorgan failure occurred in 12% of the step-up approach group compared with 40% in the open group. The step-up approach was associated with a lower incidence of incisional hernias (7% vs 24%) and new-onset diabetes (16% vs 38%) compared with the open group; however, the mortality rates did not differ between the two groups.[22]

Percutaneous

The use of percutaneous large-bore catheters for drainage is somewhat controversial. Some early studies have shown promising results, but patient selection and characterization is key. Freeny and colleagues[23] published their results of 34 subjects with necrotizing pancreatitis and medically uncontrolled sepsis treated with drainage and irrigation through large-bore catheters started a mean of 9 days after symptom onset. Of these subjects, 47% avoided an operation, 26% required immediate surgery, and 26% ultimately required delayed repair of a pancreaticocutaneous fistula. The overall mortality rate was 12%, which is comparable to the previously described open procedures. Echenique and colleagues[24] published their results of 20 subjects with necrotizing pancreatitis who were treated in a similar fashion, finding a 100% success rate with none requiring further operative interventions. These subjects differed in that they were all hemodynamically stable at time of selection, which may have contributed to their overwhelmingly positive results. Some investigators have advocated this technique only be used as a bridging procedure in unstable patients, whereas others feel that the percutaneous approach is a good tool for draining abscesses but less useful for performing extended necrosectomy.[14] As with other procedures, the risk for developing pancreaticocutaneous fistulae is significant, as high as 45% in those with disconnected duct syndrome.[25] Therefore, it may be helpful to evaluate the ductal system before implementing this technique.

Endoscopic techniques may combine transpapillary drainage with transluminal drainage. Placement of transpapillary drains, such as nasopancreatic tubes, can be used for drainage or for continuous lavage and endoscopic ultrasound (EUS)-guided transgastric or transduodenal catheter or stent placement for internal drainage of fluid or low-viscosity debris. This is followed by debridement via a gastroscope that is repeated as needed until all necrotic debris is removed, at which time the nasopancreatic tube may be removed. The stents, however, are left in place until CT evidence of resolution.[19,26,27]

An early study, published in 1997, by Baron and colleagues,[28] reported the results of 31 subjects treated in this manner, 81% of which had complete resolution and avoided an open operation. Multiple subsequent studies have demonstrated similar results, with success rates varying between 69% and 100%.[19,26] Two studies reported specifically on bleeding complications, citing an incidence of 17% to 31%.[26] The reported overall complication rates are between 7% and 25%. The largest study to date, by Seifert and colleagues,[29] included 93 subjects and reported a mortality rate of 7.5%. A retrospective study by Connor and colleagues,[30] compared the outcomes in 88 subjects treated with either endoscopic or open necrosectomy. They found that, despite a similar preoperative Acute Physiology and Chronic Health Evaluation (APACHE) II score, the open group had higher scores postoperatively. In addition, they found a trend toward increased survival in the minimally invasive surgery group ($P = .06$) along with a shorter postoperative ICU stay but longer overall hospital stay.[30]

A similar approach using a combination of transgastric or transduodenal endoscopic stent placement and percutaneous drainage is reported. The percutaneous drains are used for lavage and the transluminal stents are used for drainage. Results from a study of 15 subjects receiving this therapy demonstrated a 100% success rate with 0% mortality and no pancreaticocutaneous fistulas.[25]

Some investigators believe that, for minimally invasive techniques, endoscopic therapy may be associated with less postprocedural SIRS than is associated with open necrosectomy.[20] Direct comparisons are hard to find to validate these assertions. There are no randomized controlled trials comparing the morbidity and mortality of endoscopic techniques and open necrosectomy. Although percutaneous, endoscopic, and advanced videoscopic techniques may have use in very specific situations, there are several caveats that must be understood. All of these techniques are only as good as the people who perform them. The requisite technical expertise and judgment for many of these procedures is not widely available in all centers, let alone all geographic regions. Even when the personnel, resources, and equipment are available, biology still wins. The nature of the material that needs to be drained or be removed will be the absolute determinant of what approaches can be effectively used. Furthermore, the solution must be not only clinically effective but also cost-effective.

PERIPANCREATIC FLUID DRAINAGE

Fluid collections associated with acute pancreatitis fall into two main categories: those acute pancreatic peripancreatic fluid collections that may or may not be infected and long-standing fluid collections, such as walled-off necrosis or abscess, or pancreatic pseudocysts. A significant fluid collection is seen in 40% of hospitalized patients with acute pancreatitis who undergo CT imaging.[31] Although half of these collections spontaneously resolve, the other half may require intervention.[31] Potential complications of chronic fluid collections include rupture, infection, hemorrhage, and biliary or enteric obstruction.[32] The specific treatment depends on the cause, which may include ductal disruptions, edema, or liquefied necrosis.

The most recent update on the Atlanta Classification of peripancreatic fluid collections includes acute peripancreatic fluid collection, pseudocyst, acute necrotic collection, walled-off necrosis, and postnecrosectomy pseudocyst.[2,7] Acute peripancreatic fluid collections typically do not have connection with the ductal system and more than 50% to 70% resolve spontaneously within a few weeks.[15] The other 30% to 50% may develop into pseudocysts. Because they frequently resolve spontaneously and usually remain sterile, observation is the treatment of choice.[5,15]

An acute necrotic collection contains fluid and necrotic tissue and is found less than 4 weeks following an episode of necrotizing pancreatitis.[2,7] If this entity is mistaken for a pseudocyst there is near universal failure of any drainage procedure.[3] Instead, treatment should consist of observation and medical management unless the patient develops symptoms or the fluid collection becomes infected, in which case intervention is required.[3] In cases that require intervention, open surgical drainage is probably the gold standard,[3] although many of the same arguments that are applied to the treatment of pancreatic necrosis apply.

PSEUDOCYSTS

Pseudocysts are defined by the International Symposium on Acute Pancreatitis as "a collection of pancreatic juice enclosed by a wall of fibrous or granulation tissue which arises as a consequence of acute pancreatitis, trauma, or chronic pancreatitis."[2,7] The incidence is 5% to 16% of all new cases of acute pancreatitis.[5] They present greater than 4 weeks after the onset of symptoms and occur most commonly with interstitial edematous pancreatitis.[5] Pseudocysts are the result of direct leakage of pancreatic juice. The communication with the secretory space may spontaneously seal or remain patent, with the latter having a much lower incidence of spontaneous resolution.[15] The diagnosis of pseudocyst is confirmed with contrast-enhanced CT.[2]

Although it is not essential to delineate communication to the ductal system to secure a diagnosis, it may be helpful in predicting spontaneous resolution and in helping to direct therapy.[2,33] However, if contrast via endoscopic retrograde cholangiopancreatography (ERCP) demonstrates a communication, some investigators suggest drainage should be performed within 24 hours to prevent bacterial contamination of the pseudocyst.[17,34]

Earlier work by Bradley and colleagues,[35] published in 1979, showed that 46% of all pseudocysts will develop major complications and only 20% will spontaneously resolve. Therefore, the advice was to intervene on pseudocysts that were larger than 6 cm or those that persisted for more than 6 weeks. Mortality rates of 7% and morbidity rates of greater than 40% were reported with these operations.[33,35] It now seems that half of patients who have asymptomatic pseudocysts, regardless of size, will probably resolve spontaneously. Acute intervention is generally reserved for those patients who are symptomatic, have signs of infection, develop complications, show increasing size of the pseudocyst, or in whom it is not possible to differentiate a pseudocyst from a cystic neoplasm. In the asymptomatic patient, regardless of pseudocyst size, it is recommended to postpone intervention for at least 6 weeks to monitor for signs of resolution and to allow the wall to mature.[3,36]

Internal Drainage Procedures

The goal of drainage procedures, simply put, is to allow for controlled drainage of pancreatic juice into the lumen of the alimentary tract (preferably proximal) or to an external source (controlled pancreatic fistula).

Open internal drainage procedures were once first-line treatment of pancreatic pseudocysts.[2] They still work quite well in many situations in which other techniques fall short. Usually, they are now reserved for cases that fail less invasive options or in cases of complete obstruction of the main pancreatic duct, ductal changes associated with chronic pancreatitis, strictures, stones, or giant or multiple pseudocysts.[33] Options include Roux-en-Y pseudocyst jejunostomy, pseudocystgastrostomy, or pseudocyst duodenostomy.[2] Overall, mortality rates are reported to be 7%, whereas recurrence rates range from 5% to 20%[3] and complication rates are 12% to 24%.[2,4] However, the corresponding author thinks many practitioners would consider those rates to be on the high end for well-selected patients.

Percutaneous internal drainage can be done with the assistance of either ultrasound or CT guidance. Most commonly, the anterior abdominal wall, the anterior gastric wall, and the posterior gastric wall are punctured with a needle to gain entry into the pseudocyst. This is then exchanged over a guidewire for a double-J, 5F to10F catheter that drains the pseudocyst into the stomach.[4] Because treatment failures are higher, percutaneous internal drainage is reserved for patients who are poor candidates for operative or other more definitive treatment or as a temporary measure in patients with infected pseudocysts.[4] The risk of developing pancreaticocutaneous fistulae and drain tract or pseudocyst infections is increased with percutaneous techniques compared with open internal drainage.[4]

Endoscopic internal drainage has excellent outcomes that, in many cases, are similar to operative management but with perhaps less procedural morbidity.[4] However, there are no randomized controlled trials directly comparing the two.[34] Despite the lack of comparative trials, seven published guidelines recommend endoscopic therapy as the initial treatment of uncomplicated pseudocysts.[37,38] The endoscopic approach may also require multiple endoscopic attempts and repeated imaging studies, which will influence comparative cost and risk.

Endoscopic drainage seems to be associated with a learning curve as evidenced by increasing rates of pseudocyst resolution from 45% to 93% with endoscopists who have performed more than 20 procedures.[2,34] Transpapillary access is used when there is demonstrable ductal communication with the pseudocyst.[4] A 5F or 7F stent is then placed into the pancreatic duct and either directly into the cyst or used to bridge the leak.[2] This is left in place until there is CT evidence of resolution.[3] Biliary and pancreatic sphincterotomies are also performed.[4] If no ductal communication can be demonstrated, transluminal access may be used via a transgastric or medial duodenal wall approach.[32] EUS may be helpful when there is no visible bulge into the lumen. EUS may also identify the distance between the viscera and the pseudocyst, intervening vessels, the thickness of the cyst wall, or the presence of necrosis, which may alter management in up to 20% of patients.[4] Once the pseudocyst is identified, contrast injection is performed to confirm placement of the needle and enterotomy and pseudocystotomy are made to allow passage of a guidewire followed by placement of one or two 7F to 10F stents.[4] Stents are left in place for several months or until radiographic resolution.[3,4] Reported success rates vary from 82% to 100%[2] with decreasing success rates as the pseudocyst location moves from the head to the body to the tail of the pancreas.[4] Recurrence rates range from 5% to 20%.[4] Overall complication rates are as high as 34% and consist of hemorrhage, perforation, infection, stent migration or occlusion, or recurrent pancreatitis.[2,4]

Disadvantages of this approach are that the stents are fairly small, thus the cyst must be minimally loculated, nonviscous, and contain little or no debris. Also, in cases of diagnostic insecurity, there is limited ability to obtain a cyst wall biopsy.[4,17] Necrosis is associated with a 50% failure rate and increased rates of recurrence and complications. Treatment in patients with necrosis should probably be surgical.[4]

Laparoscopic approaches seem, thus far, to have similar results to open procedures. However, there are no prospective controlled trials comparing the two. In reviewing all large series (n ≥10) of laparoscopic internal drainage (total of 89 subjects), 10.1% required conversion to an open procedure, 6.7% had bleeding complications, 5.6% developed sepsis, 3.4% had a recurrence, 4.5% required an additional procedure, and the mortality rate was 1.1%.[4]

Pseudocystgastrostomy may be created via either an anterior or a posterior approach.[4] For either open or videoscopic approach, the techniques for pseudocystgastrostomy are similar. The anterior approach involves making an anterior gastrotomy, then identifying the point of maximal bulge on the posterior wall signifying the pseudocyst location. A needle is then used to confirm this. A biopsy of the pseudocyst wall may be obtained to rule out malignancy when clinical suspicion is present. Pseudocystgastrostomy is made with either a stapler or sutures followed by closure of the anterior gastrotomy. A similar anterior approach has been described using two to three balloon-tipped trocars placed into the peritoneum and then directly through the anterior stomach via separate 10 mm gastrotomies. The balloons are then inflated and the anterior stomach wall is compressed to the abdominal wall such that the remainder of the procedure can be performed without traversing the peritoneum. A minilaparoscopic technique uses 2 mm instruments placed directly into the gastric lumen using endoscopic guidance, thus avoiding the need for pneumoperitoneum. However, 10% require conversion due to inability to localize the pseudocyst.[4]

The posterior or lesser sac approach was developed to avoid the technical challenges of the anterior approach and to avoid an additional gastrotomy. The lesser sac is accessed by dividing the greater omentum along the greater curve of the stomach. The proponents of this technique suggest there is better visualization and improved ability to locate the pseudocyst without the need for a visible bulge in the gastric wall. In addition, there is less bleeding and a larger anastomosis resulting in improved patency rates.[4] The corresponding author does not recommend this technique because the inflammatory process frequently obliterates the lesser sac and this approach may convert a contained situation into a diffuse intraabdominal process.

Drainage via pseudocyst jejunostomy may be preferable if the pseudocyst is not in close proximity to the stomach or duodenum. The pseudocyst may be anastomosed to a Roux-en-Y jejunal limb. The pseudocyst is entered via the transverse mesocolon or through the gastrocolic ligament. One small study evaluating eight subjects using this approach demonstrated no conversions, complications, or recurrences at 2 years.[4]

External Drainage Procedures

External drainage may be necessary when there is evidence of gross infection of the pseudocyst or in situations in which the pseudocyst wall is too thin to use for a secure anastomosis.[17] These procedures generally result in a pancreatic fistula, which is fine as long as it is controlled.

Open external drainage has become extremely uncommon due to high morbidity but may be considered in complex situations.[4] Percutaneous drainage can be performed via a retroperitoneal or transperitoneal approach.[31] A transgastric approach may also be used; however, it is associated with an increased risk for infecting a previously sterile fluid collection; therefore, it should only be considered when other options are less available. Aspiration alone has recurrence rates of greater than 70% and should not be used.[31] Drains are typically left in place for 3 weeks but can be required for as long as several months or longer if ductal communication is present.[17] Once drain output has decreased to a low volume per day and imaging shows no persistent fluid collection, sinography may be performed to evaluate for resolution of the pseudocyst, persistence of ductal communication, retained debris, or presence of a pseudocyst enteric fistula.[31] Potential complications of percutaneous drainage include bleeding (1%–2%), transversal of the pleural space or other viscera (1%–2%), and chronic pancreaticocutaneous fistula (5%).[31] The risk of developing a pancreaticocutaneous fistula increases when persistent ductal communication is present.[3] Reported success rates are variable, ranging from 60% to 100%.[4,31,34]

D'Egidio and Schein[39] evaluated the success of percutaneous drainage based on a proposed ductal classification system. Type 1 ducts have normal anatomy and rare communication with the pseudocyst, type 2 ducts have a diseased pancreatic duct without stricture but often with duct-pseudocyst communication, and type 3 ducts have stricture and pseudocyst communication. In their study, subjects with type 1 ducts showed resolution with drainage in all 13 cases, those with type 2 ducts achieved resolution in 9 of 10 cases, and those with type 3 ducts were excluded. Zhang and colleagues[40] also reported outcomes based on D'Egidio classifications and found a success rate of 82% for type 1 ducts, 60% for type 2, and again excluded type 3 ducts.

Most published literature comparing percutaneous external drainage to open external drainage report a higher mortality, longer length of stay, and higher incidence of complications with percutaneous drainage. The only prospective study comparing percutaneous with open drainage found resolution rates of 93% with open drainage and 75% with percutaneous drainage.[4] The data seem to suggest that percutaneous drainage should be reserved for patients with normal ducts who are not candidates for operative management or as a temporizing measure until more definitive measures can be used. It is also a valid option for infected pseudocysts if there is no associated necrosis.[2,15,33,37]

Resection

Resection of the pseudocyst with associated segmental pancreatectomy should be performed in cases in which it is impossible to differentiate a pseudocyst from a malignant cystic neoplasm[33] or for patients in whom the acute inflammatory process has long since resolved and the morbidity of the pancreatic resection is less than that of a drainage procedure. Most frequently, this is in the case of pseudocysts located in the very distal portion of the tail or in patients who develop a disconnected pancreatic tail syndrome.[17,33] If the pseudocyst is near the spleen or involves the splenic vessels, it may be necessary to perform concomitant splenectomy.[33]

WALLED-OFF NECROSIS

Walled-off necrosis differs from pancreatic necrosis because it is typically associated with a limited degree of necrosis, a more clinically benign course, and mortality rates of 5%. It is also rare, comprising less than 5% of all peripancreatic fluid collections.[2,17] Walled-off necrosis represents the mature encapsulated form of an acute necrotic collection that usually develops more than 4 weeks after the initial episode of acute necrotizing pancreatitis. Walled-off necrosis now includes the former entities described as organized pancreatic necrosis, pancreatic pseudocyst with necrosis, pancreatic sequestrum, necroma, and subacute pancreatic necrosis.[6] The diagnosis is made by CT demonstrating an encapsulated peripancreatic collection of solid and fluid debris in the correct clinical context and infection is confirmed with fine-needle aspiration demonstrating organisms.[8] Walled-off necrosis can be sterile or infected and may or may not be in communication with the ductal system.[2] The treatment includes drainage and antibiotics until radiographic evidence of resolution.[2,3,8] Open drainage or debridement has been the most common form of treatment. The addition of continuous postoperative lavage and open packing with debridement repeated every 2 to 4 days has decreased mortality in some cases.[15] If the necrosis is well delineated, it may be possible to perform only one operation for debridement with drains for postoperative irrigation.[15] The optimal timing for open drainage is 3 to 4 weeks after the onset to allow for demarcation and additional improvement in mortality,[2] as well as to decrease the need for subsequent operation.

Percutaneous drainage may be acceptable when there is no surrounding necrosis, the collection is well localized and there is no communication with the ductal system. The success rate with this approach approximates 90% with appropriate patient selection. It can also be used as a bridge to open drainage if the fluid collection has been present fewer than 4 weeks since the onset of symptoms.[2,17] Laparoscopic and endoscopic techniques may be equally as effective as surgery.[2]

DUCTAL DISRUPTIONS

In patients in whom main pancreatic ductal disruption is suspected, it is imperative to clearly define the ductal anatomy to the best degree possible.[41] Imaging with CT may suggest the site of the leak based on fluid location and may also yield information about ductal dilatation that may be important in determining optimal management.[2]

Significant ductal disruptions will result in internal fistula, external fistula, pancreatic pleural effusion, pancreatic ascites, or disconnected pancreatic tail syndrome. Although these sound like a collection of entities, they are more likely just a continuum of the same pathophysiologic process with different resolutions.

Internal fistulae are uncommon and are the result of ductal disruptions that are not contained by the inflammatory response. The location of the ductal disruption corresponds to the location of the fluid collection with anterior ductal disruptions resulting in pancreatic ascites and posterior disruptions resulting in pancreatic pleural effusions.[41] Once it is confirmed that a large fluid collection in either the chest or peritoneal cavity is pancreatic enzyme rich, the diagnosis is secure. Management begins with percutaneous external drainage to covert the clinical picture to that of a controlled fistula. This alone may result in spontaneous closure in 70% to 82% of cases.[41] It can also serve as a temporary measure until later definitive management can be done.[12,41] After percutaneous drainage, endoscopic retrograde pancreatography (ERP) with papillary decompression via sphincterotomy or transpapillary stenting should be performed to decrease the resistance to flow of pancreatic juice into the duodenum.[41] More definitive operative intervention will most likely be required in situations such as the inability to cannulate the duct, multiple ductal strictures are present, the duct has a large defect, or there is a disconnected duct.[41] Dilated ducts (main pancreatic duct measuring greater than 7 mm) may be treated with lateral pancreaticojejunostomy with relatively low morbidity and mortality rates.[41]

If the ducts are small, the specific site of duct disruption becomes more important in directing management.[41] If the disruption is in the tail, a caudal pancreatectomy may be a better solution.[41] If the disruption is in the body, a distal pancreatectomy plus or minus concomitant splenectomy may be performed.[41]

If the ductal disruption is in the head of the pancreas, matters become more challenging. The solution may require a pancreatic head resection or operative conversion to internal drainage. The reported success rates range from 77% to 100% and long-term failure rates are due to obliteration of the fistula tract.[41] All of these management options can be very challenging and correct choice of procedure, as well as correct choice of timing of intervention, are mandatory for success. Very experienced teams should do all of these operations.

External fistulae are typically the result of a percutaneous drain placed for pseudocyst treatment.[41] The chance of developing this complication is greater if there is also a stricture or obstruction of the main pancreatic duct resulting in ductal hypertension.[41] Other causes include previous operative therapy such as necrosectomy, pancreatic resection, or pancreatic injury during splenectomy or nephrectomy.[41] Treatment involves ERP with sphincterotomy and stenting, which results in fistula closure in 40% to 90%.[41–43]

The location of the leak may give insight into the chance of closure without operative intervention. Howard and colleagues[44] found spontaneous closure with conservative therapy in 87% of postoperative side fistulas compared with 53% of inflammatory side fistulas and 0% of end fistulas. Better results are seen in side fistulas that can be bridged with a stent, with 92% to 100% resolving without an operation.[42] At least 6 weeks should be allowed for ductal disruptions to heal before any further intervention is undertaken unless the main pancreatic duct is dilated, in which case the fistula is unlikely to heal and operative intervention is the treatment of choice.[41] The operation is determined by the location of the ductal disruption, as stated above. Despite operative therapy, recurrence of the pancreaticocutaneous fistula occurs in 23% of cases.[9] A more detailed description of the management of pancreatic fistulae is found by Hardacre and colleagues elsewhere in this issue.

Disconnected pancreatic tail syndrome is perhaps the most common variant of an inflammatory fistula and develops in 16% of patients with a pancreatic fluid collection and/or fistula.[12] A high index of suspicion should be present in cases of recurrent pseudocysts or persistent fistulae.[12] Initial work-up should include exclusion of vascular abnormalities such as pseudoaneurysm or splenic vein thrombosis.[9] Management options are similar to those mentioned above, including long-term stenting, endoscopic transluminal drainage, transpapillary drainage, surgical drainage via pseudocystgastrostomy, pseudocyst enterostomy, or side-to-side pancreaticojejunostomy of the upstream pancreas to a Roux-en-y limb, or resection, including left-sided pancreatectomy with or without splenectomy and the Whipple procedure.[9,10,12] Endoscopic drainage is preferred initially because recurrence rates are high but equal to operative drainage results.[9]

ASSOCIATED OPERATIONS AND PROCEDURES
Biliary Procedures

Early studies demonstrated that ERCP with endoscopic sphincterotomy (ES) may reduce morbidity in acute pancreatitis but has no effect on mortality. This reduction in morbidity is due to decreasing the impact of biliary sepsis and not because removing the stone decreases the evolution of pancreatitis.[18] In 2002, the International Association of Pancreatology (IAP) released evidence-based guidelines regarding ERCP and ES in the management of gallstone pancreatitis, stating that these interventions are indicated in cases of obstructive jaundice and cholangitis.[16] The 2007 American Gastroenterology Association guidelines state that ERCP and ES should only be used for treatment of cholangitis.[16]

The role of prophylactic biliary procedures is less clear. In patients who develop pancreatitis as the result of gallstones, the source of the gallstones must be addressed given an overall recurrence rate of biliary pancreatitis of 29% to 63%.[16] However, the debate continues in regard to the optimal timing at which cholecystectomy is performed. An early study by Kelly and Wagner, in 1988, assigned 165 subjects to cholecystectomy before or after 48 hours. They found a much higher morbidity and mortality in the early cholecystectomy group compared with the late group (83% vs 48% and 18% vs 12%, respectively).[45] In 2012, van Baal and colleagues[46] conducted a systematic review that included 998 subjects, 48% of whom had a cholecystectomy during their index admission and 52% had an interval cholecystectomy at a median of 40 days. They found a statistically significant increase in complications in the interval cholecystectomy group, with 18% requiring readmission, 8% developing recurrent biliary pancreatitis, 3% developing acute cholecystitis, and 7% requiring readmission for biliary colic. This is in contrast to those who had a cholecystectomy during their index hospitalization, in which none suffered any recurrent biliary events. They also found the overall conversion from laparoscopic to open to be 7%, with no significant difference between the groups. Sinha and colleagues[47] concluded that interval cholecystectomy resulted in more frequent difficult dissection of the Calot triangle compared with index cholecystectomy in 42% versus 12% cases, respectively. The main problem with the published reports on this topic is the variation in practice and the extreme range of timing options evaluated.

The IAP recommends that, in mild gallstone pancreatitis, cholecystectomy should be performed as soon as the patient recovers and, ideally, this should be done in the same hospitalization. In severe cases, they recommend delaying surgery until there is sufficient resolution of the inflammation and clinical recovery. In addition, they state that to reduce the risk of recurrence endoscopic sphincterotomy is an alternative to cholecystectomy in patients who are not fit for surgery.[16]

Vascular Complications

Vascular complications affect approximately 2.4% to 10% of patients with pancreatitis and include pseudoaneurysms and bleeding from erosion into an artery.[48] The most frequently involved vessels are the splenic, gastroduodenal, pancreaticoduodenal, and the left gastric arteries.[48] These may rupture into the peritoneal cavity or into the gastrointestinal tract, which is accompanied by mortality rates of approximately 50%.[48] In the past, operative management was the mainstay of therapy though fraught with great difficulty. Advances in interventional radiographic techniques have made embolization the preferred management.[48] Radiological management has been proven to be effective and reliable in both elective and emergency treatment of arterial complications of pancreatitis.[48] In patients with hemorrhage into pseudocysts, a combined approach should be used that begins with hemorrhage control by angiographic means followed by treatment of the pseudocyst as required.[48]

Colonic Complications

Colonic complications of acute pancreatitis are uncommon, occurring in approximately 1% of cases, but can be associated with a very poor prognosis despite surgical intervention.[49] The most common manifestation is colonic ileus, which is not life threatening. Sustained ileus may, however, necessitate the need for prolonged parenteral nutritional support, which is attended by potential complication. The more grave forms of colonic complications are obstruction, necrosis, perforation, and fistulae. Obstruction may occur from either extrinsic compression by a pancreatic inflammatory mass or fluid collection or from pericolonic fibrosis. The most common site of stenosis is the splenic flexure, which may be due relatively poor arterial supply and close proximity to the tail of the pancreas. Colonic necrosis and perforation are potentially lethal complications, with an overall mortality of 58%.[49] The most common locations are the transverse colon and splenic flexure with pancreatic necrosis and abscess with vascular compromise being the most common inciting events. The surgical management remains difficult and includes resection of the involved colon and exteriorization with either a proximal colostomy or ileostomy and a distal mucous fistula. The decision to resect is based on surgical experience and adherence to fundamental surgical principles because there are few guidelines to assist with management decisions.[49]

SUMMARY

The operative management of acute pancreatitis is focused on managing the acute complications, the long-term sequelae, or the prevention of recurrent pancreatitis. Using the least amount of intervention to achieve the stated goals has always been the case. However, the evolution of videoscopic and endoscopic techniques have greatly expanded the tools available. Patience, vigilance, expertise, and judgment, and an ability to be humbled are necessary for the successful practitioner who manages patients with severe pancreatitis.

REFERENCES

1. Baron TH, Morgan DE. Acute necrotizing pancreatitis. N Engl J Med 1999; 340(18):1412-7.
2. Brun A, Agarwal N, Pitchumoni CS. Fluid collections in and around the pancreas in acute pancreatitis. J Clin Gastroenterol 2011;45(7):614-23.
3. Baron TH, Morgan DE. The diagnosis and management of fluid collections associated with the pancreas. Am J Med 1997;102:555-63.
4. Berman S, Melvin S. Operative and nonoperative management of pancreatic pseudocysts. Surg Clin North Am 2007;87:1447-60.
5. Bollen TL. Imaging of acute pancreatitis: update of the revised Atlanta classification. Radiol Clin North Am 2012;50:429-45.
6. Bollen TL, Besselink MG, van Santvoort HC, et al. Toward an update of the Atlanta classification on acute pancreatitis. Pancreas 2007;35(2):107-11.
7. Bollen TL, van Santvoort HC, Besselink MG, et al. Update on acute pancreatitis: ultrasound, computed tomography, and magnetic resonance imaging features. Semin Ultrasound CT MR 2007;28:371-83.
8. Stamatakos M, Stefanaki C, Kontzoglou K, et al. Walled-off pancreatic necrosis. World J Gastroenterol 2010;16(14):1707-12.
9. Lawrence C, Howell DA, Stefan AM, et al. Disconnected pancreatic tail syndrome: potential for endoscopic therapy and results of long-term follow-up. Gastrointest Endosc 2008;67(4):673-9.
10. Traverso WL, Kozarek RA. Interventional management of peripancreatic fluid collections. Surg Clin North Am 1999;79(4):745-57.
11. Traverso LW, Kozarek RA. Pancreatic necrosectomy: definitions and technique. J Gastrointest Surg 2005;9(3):436-9.
12. Solanki R, Koganti SB, Bheerappa N, et al. Disconnected duct syndrome: refractory inflammatory external fistula following percutaneous drainage of an infected peripancreatic fluid collection. A case report and review of the literature. JOP 2011;12(2):177-80.
13. Cappell MS. Acute pancreatitis: etiology, clinical presentation, diagnosis, and therapy. Med Clin North Am 2008;92:889-923.

14. Schneider L, Buchler MW, Werner J. Acute pancreatitis with an emphasis on infection. Infect Dis Clin North Am 2010;24:921–41.
15. Farthmann EH, Lausen M, Schoffel U. Indications for surgical treatment of acute pancreatitis. Hepatogastroenterology 1993;40:556–62.
16. Uhl W, Warshaw A, Imrie C, et al. IAP guidelines for the surgical management of acute pancreatitis. Pancreatology 2002;2:565–73.
17. Tsiotos GG, Sarr MG. Management of fluid collections and necrosis in acute pancreatitis. Curr Gastroenterol Rep 1999;1:139–44.
18. Clancy T, Ashley S. Current management of necrotizing pancreatitis. Adv Surg 2002;36:103–21.
19. Voermans RP, Veldkamp MC, Rauws EA, et al. Endoscopic transmural debridement of symptomatic organized pancreatic necrosis. Gastrointest Endosc 2007;66(5):909–16.
20. Warner EA, Ben-David K, Cendan JC. Laparoscopic pancreatic surgery: what now and what next? Curr Gastroenterol Rep 2009;11:128–33.
21. van Santvoort HC, Besselink MG, Bollen TL, et al. Casematched comparison of the retroperitoneal approach with laparotomy for necrotizing pancreatitis. World J Surg 2007;31:1635–42.
22. Van Santvoort HC, Besselink MG, Bakker OJ, et al. A step-up approach or open necrosectomy for necrotizing pancreatitis. N Engl J Med 2010;362(16):1491–502.
23. Freeny PC, Hauptmann E, Althaus SJ, et al. Percutaneous CT-guided catheter drainage of infected acute necrotizing pancreatitis: techniques and results. Am J Roentgenol 1998;170:969.
24. Echenique AM, Sleeman D, Yrizarry J, et al. Percutaneous catheter-directed debridement of infected pancreatic necrosis: results in 20 patients. J Vasc Interv Radiol 1998;9:565.
25. Ross A, Gluck M, Irani S, et al. Combined endoscopic and percutaneous drainage of organized pancreatic necrosis. Gastrointest Endosc 2010;71(1):79–84.
26. Friedland S, Kaltenbach T, Sugimoto M, et al. Endoscopic necrosectomy of organized pancreatic necrosis: a currently practiced NOTES procedure. J Hepatobiliary Pancreat Surg 2009;16:266–9.
27. Ho HS, Frey CF. Gastrointestinal and pancreatic complications associated with severe pancreatitis. Arch Surg 1995;130:817–22.
28. Baron TH, Morgan DE. Organized pancreatic necrosis: definition, diagnosis, and management. Gastroenterol Int 1997;10:167–78.
29. Seifert H, Biermer M, Schmitt W, et al. Transluminal endoscopic necrosectomy after acute pancreatitis: a multicenter study with long-term follow-up (The GEPARD Study). Gut 2009;58:1260.
30. Connor S, Alexakis N, Raraty MG, et al. Early and late complications after pancreatic necrosectomy. Surgery 2005;137:499–505.
31. Neff R. Pancreatic pseudocysts and fluid collections—percutaneous approaches. Surg Clin North Am 2001;81(2):399–403.
32. Kozarek RA, Ball TJ, Patterson DJ, et al. Endoscopic transpapillary therapy for disrupted pancreatic duct and peripancreatic fluid collections. Gastroenterology 1991;100:1362–70.
33. Behrns KE, Ben-David K. Surgical therapy of pancreatic pseudocysts. J Gastrointest Surg 2008;12:2231–9.
34. Cannon JW, Callery MP, Vollmer CM. Diagnosis and management of pancreatic pseudocysts: what is the evidence? J Am Coll Surg 2009;209(3):385–93.
35. Bradley EL, Clements JL, Gonzalez AC. The natural history of pancreatic pseudocysts: a unified concept of management. Am J Surg 1979;137(1):135–41.

36. Nealon WH, Bawduniak J, Walser EM. Appropriate timing of cholecystectomy in patients who present with moderate to severe gallstone-associated acute pancreatitis with peripancreatic fluid collections. Ann Surg 2004;239(6):741–51.
37. Loveday BP, Mittal A, Phillips A, et al. Minimally invasive management of pancreatic abscess, pseudocyst, and necrosis: a systematic review of current guidelines. World J Surg 2008;32:2382–94.
38. Martin RF, Marion MD. Resectional therapy for chronic pancreatitis. Surg Clin North Am 2007;87:1461–75.
39. D'Egidio A, Schein M. Percutaneous drainage of pancreatic pseudocysts: A prospective study. World J Surg 1991;16:141.
40. Zhang AB, Zheng SS. Treatment of pancreatic pseudocysts in line with D'Egidio's classification. World J Gastroenterol 2005;11(5):729–32.
41. Morgan KA, Adams DB. Management of internal and external pancreatic fistulas. Surg Clin North Am 2007;87:1503–13.
42. Rana SS, Bhasin DK, Nanda M, et al. Endoscopic transpapillary drainage for external fistulas developing after surgical or radiological pancreatic interventions. J Gastroenterol Hepatol 2010;25:1087–92.
43. Ranson JH. The role of surgery in the management of acute pancreatitis. Ann Surg 1990;211(4):382–93.
44. Howard TJ, Stonerock CE, Sarkar J, et al. Contemporary treatment strategies for external pancreatic fistulas. Surgery 1998;124:627–32.
45. Kelly TR, Wagner DS. Gallstone pancreatitis: A prospective randomized trial of the timing of surgery. Surgery 1988;104:600–5.
46. van Baal M, Besselink MG, Bakker OJ, et al. Timing of cholecystectomy after mild biliary pancreatitis. Ann Surg 2012;255(5):860–6.
47. Sinha R. Early laparoscopic cholecystectomy in acute biliary pancreatitis: the optimal choice? HPB (Oxford) 2008;10:332–5.
48. Sawlani V, Phadke RV, Baijal SS, et al. Arterial complications of pancreatitis and their radiological management. Australas Radiol 1996;40:381–6.
49. Aldridge MC, Francis ND, Glazer G, et al. Colonic complications of severe acute pancreatitis. Br J Surg 1989;76:362–7.

Management of Pancreatic Fistulas

Jeffrey A. Blatnik, MD, Jeffrey M. Hardacre, MD*

KEYWORDS

• Pancreatic fistula • Management • Therapy

KEY POINTS

- A pancreatic fistula is defined as the leakage of pancreatic fluid as a result of pancreatic duct disruption; such ductal disruptions may be either iatrogenic or noniatrogenic.
- The management of pancreatic fistulas can be complex and mandates a multidisciplinary approach.
- Basic principles of fistula control/patient stabilization, delineation of ductal anatomy, and definitive therapy remain of paramount importance.

INTRODUCTION AND DEFINITION

Pancreatic fistula is a well-recognized complication of pancreatic surgery and pancreatitis. Successful management of this potentially complex problem often requires a multidisciplinary approach. A pancreatic fistula is defined as the leakage of pancreatic fluid as a result of pancreatic duct disruption. Such ductal disruptions may be either iatrogenic or noniatrogenic. Noniatrogenic fistulas typically result from either acute or chronic pancreatitis, caused most frequently by gallstones or alcohol.

Iatrogenic pancreatic fistulas usually result from operative trauma, which typically occurs in the tail of the pancreas during splenic surgery, during left renal/adrenal surgery, or during mobilization of the splenic flexure of the colon. More frequently, pancreatic fistulas occur following resection of a portion of the pancreas. For postoperative pancreatic fistulas, a consensus definition and grading scale were developed to aide in their classification.[1] The definition of a postoperative pancreatic fistula is drain output of any volume on or after postoperative day 3 with an amylase greater than 3 times the serum level. Iatrogenic fistulas may also result from complications of endoscopic interventions during endoscopic retrograde cholangiopancreatography (ERCP).

A pancreatic fistula can drain to either an internal or an external location. An internal pancreatic fistula is usually seen in patients with a history of pancreatitis, in which the

Department of Surgery, Case Western Reserve University, University Hospitals Case Medical Center, 11100 Euclid Avenue, Cleveland, OH 44106, USA
* Corresponding author.
E-mail address: Jeffrey.Hardacre@UHhospitals.org

Surg Clin N Am 93 (2013) 611–617
http://dx.doi.org/10.1016/j.suc.2013.02.011
0039-6109/13/$ – see front matter © 2013 Elsevier Inc. All rights reserved.

leakage is not controlled by the inflammatory response. Such fistulas may manifest as pancreatic ascites or a pancreaticopleural fistula. An external pancreatic fistula can also be called a pancreaticocutaneous fistula. These fistulas often occur after percutaneous drainage of a pancreatic fluid collection/pseudocyst, following pancreatic debridement, or after a pancreatic resection.

Regardless of the cause or location of the pancreatic fistula, the steps required for treatment are similar. First, stabilization of patients and medical optimization are crucial. Controlling the fistula, controlling sepsis, and providing adequate nutrition typically accomplish this. Second, the area of pancreatic duct injury must be identified. Finally, definitive management of the fistula should be addressed.

INITIAL MANAGEMENT

The first step in the management of patients with a pancreatic fistula is control of the pancreatic secretions. This step is accomplished with percutaneous drains placed under computed tomography (CT) or ultrasound guidance. Drainage of fluid collections along with antibiotics when appropriate help control the inflammation and potential source of infection. Following control of the fluid, the next step is to medically optimize patients. Patients with a pancreatic fistula are at risk for having significant nutritional and electrolyte imbalances. Particularly, patients have significant loss of sodium and bicarbonate caused by pancreatic exocrine secretions. Nutritionally, patients with pancreatic fistulas often present with significant nausea, anorexia, and the inability to tolerate oral intake. In addition, pending the severity of the pancreatic fistula, these patients often have poor nutritional absorption, particularly of protein and fat. Given this, patients may require total parenteral nutrition (TPN) in an effort to overcome their catabolic state. TPN provides the benefit of minimizing protein loss while ideally minimizing pancreatic enzyme secretion. TPN, however, is not without risks to patients, including potential line sepsis and cholestatic injury to the liver. With this in mind, enteral feeding should be initiated when possible because it is relatively simple to administer, less costly than TPN, and has the ability to maintain mucosal barrier function. Ideally, this would be postpyloric in nature via a nasojejunal feeding tube. However, the benefits of postpyloric feeding over gastric feeding are debatable.[2]

EVALUATING THE PANCREATIC DUCT

Following stabilization of patients, the next step in management is to identify the location and extent of pancreatic duct injury. This information can help dictate the need for additional interventional procedures and will be vital in creating operative plans should patients require surgical intervention. At this point in the management of patients with a pancreatic fistula, a CT has surely been done to asses for and drain any fluid collections. To evaluate the pancreatic duct magnetic resonance cholangiopancreatography (MRCP) and ERCP are used. MRCP is noninvasive and delineates the sites of ductal disruption as well as other findings, such as stones or strictures. A supplement to standard MRCP includes secretin stimulation MRCP, which is useful in the diagnosis of chronic pancreatitis by stressing the pancreas to produce exocrine secretions while performing the imaging. Regardless of the type of MRCP, it remains only a diagnostic modality. In contrast, ERCP has the benefit of visualizing the pancreatic duct while at the same time providing potentially therapeutic interventions, including sphincterotomy, stenting, and nasobiliary drainage. ERCP, however, requires conscious sedation and carries the risk of duodenal perforation (<1.0%) or pancreatitis (3.5%).[3] Finally, in patients who have already undergone percutaneous drainage, a fistulogram can be performed through the drain as a simple method to visualize the area of pancreatic ductal injury.

DEFINITIVE MANAGEMENT OF THE PANCREATIC FISTULA

After the anatomy of the pancreatic duct and the location of the injury have been identified, attention can be turned toward definitive management of the fistula. It should be noted, that 70% to 82% of pancreatic fistulas will close spontaneously without the need for operative intervention.[4,5] Often, simply making patients nil per os (NPO) and reducing pancreatic stimulation will, over time, result in resolution of the pancreatic fistula. However, there are certain pancreatic fistulas that will eventually require intervention.

Octreotide

Octreotide, a synthetic somatostatin analogue inhibits pancreatic exocrine secretion. It is commonly thought that octreotide facilitates spontaneous fistula closure. However, a meta-analysis evaluating octreotide failed to show any improvement in the rate of fistula closure.[6] Despite the lack of effect on fistula closure rate, octreotide may help lower fistula output and make fistula control easier.

Fibrin Glue

Fibrin glue has been used to obliterate the fistula tract. This technique involves injection of fibrin glue either under radiographic guidance or through a previously placed drainage tract. Studies of this technique are limited; but in small case series, it has been shown to be a successful treatment option for patients with low-output pancreatic fistulas.[4,7]

Endoscopic Therapy

The use of ERCP in the evaluation of a pancreatic fistula is beneficial in that it has both diagnostic and therapeutic utility. In patients with a persistent pancreatic fistula despite percutaneous drainage and medical optimization, an ERCP with sphincterotomy or stenting can be performed. This practice serves to reduce the pressure within the pancreatic duct, ideally facilitating the closure of the pancreatic fistula. In the literature, closure rates as high as 82% have been reported.[5] However, a recent multicenter series comparing endoscopic transpapillary stenting versus conservative treatment failed to show a significant improvement in the fistula closure rate (84% vs 75%) or in the time to closure (71 days vs 120 days).[8] Despite these findings, endoscopic stenting may be useful in the management of select pancreatic fistulas.

Patients who present with pancreatic ductal disruption (either complete or partial) can often be managed with an endoscopic stent to bridge the disruption with a success rate of more than 50%. Predictors of success include the ability to bridge the disruption and patients with a partial disruption.[9]

Operative Management

The operative management of pancreatic fistulas remains an important component of their treatment but is generally reserved for patients in which efforts at conservative or endoscopic procedures have failed. Surgery is often needed in patients who are unable to have endoscopic therapies secondary to postsurgical anatomy or who have an inability to cannulate the pancreatic duct, a significant ductal stricture, or a very large defect. The type of surgical intervention proposed for patients varies greatly on the location of the ductal injuries.

Patients who present with a large pancreatic duct (7 mm or greater) are generally best managed with duct decompression, usually via a lateral pancreaticojejunostomy. If a pancreatic pseudocyst is present, this area should be incorporated into the anastomosis, although frequently duct decompression alone is sufficient enough to allow resolution of the cyst.[10]

For those patients without a dilated pancreatic duct, knowing the location of the ductal injury becomes vital in preoperative planning. For example, patients with an injury isolated to the body or tail of the pancreas are often best served by a distal pancreatectomy, resecting only the area of the pancreas beyond the disruption.

Disconnected duct syndrome is a phenomenon often seen in patients following acute pancreatic necrosis in which a portion of the pancreas has undergone autolysis. Initial management is similar with supportive care and management with percutaneous drainage. Definitive management will depend on the location of the ductal disruption. If the injury is located near the tail of the pancreas, it can frequently be managed with distal pancreatectomy. If the ductal disruption is near the neck of the pancreas, then these patients are best served by draining the fistula for a period of time until a fibrous fistula tract can develop. At that time, a fistula enterostomy can be performed using a Roux-en-y jejunal limb. The success rate has been reported to be as high as 100% in certain series, with minimal comorbidities.[11] However, long-term failure may occur because of obliteration of the fistula tract over time. Another surgical option for a disconnected duct at the neck of the gland is distal pancreatectomy, but that sacrifices a notable amount of otherwise functional pancreatic parenchyma. Finally, recent studies have investigated the role of endoscopic therapies for the management of disconnected duct syndrome. Some have found that patients temporarily improved with endoscopic therapy but will often go on to require surgical intervention.[12] In patients who may not be considered a surgical candidate, or who refuse surgery, a rendezvous technique using endoscopic and percutaneous techniques may provide an alternative treatment method.[13]

TREATMENT OF POSTPROCEDURE PANCREATIC FISTULA

Postprocedural pancreatic fistulas often follow percutaneous drainage of a pancreatic pseudocyst, operative debridement of acute pancreatitis, operative pancreatic injury, or planned pancreatic resection. The management of the fistula is variable pending the cause of the fistula.

Pancreatic Fistula Associated with Pseudocyst Drainage

A pancreatic fistula following percutaneous drainage of a pseudocyst occurs approximately 15% of the time. Persistent drainage is often the result of a stricture within the main pancreatic duct, which is causing the pressure within the duct to be abnormally high. In this setting, early ERCP evaluation should be sought because the addition of a sphincterotomy or stent to reduce the pressure within the pancreatic duct will often result in spontaneous closure of the fistula. If after 6 weeks patients continue to have active drainage, then the need for operative intervention should be discussed with patients.

Pancreatic Fistula After Debridement of Pancreatic Necrosis

Patients with pancreatic necrosis secondary to acute pancreatitis often present with pancreatic duct disruption. At the time of the initial surgery, the goal is to debride all necrotic tissue and perform wide drainage. Surprisingly, many duct disruptions will go on to seal with time and drainage. However, should patients continue to have ongoing fistula drainage, then the next step will be to study the pancreatic duct anatomy. If patients can tolerate ERCP, then it should be used for decompression of the pancreatic duct. If despite ductal decompression patients still have a persistent pancreatic fistula, then operative intervention should be considered.

Pancreatic Fistula After Operative Trauma

Pancreatic fistula after operative trauma is usually isolated to the tail of the pancreas following splenectomy, left nephrectomy/adrenalectomy, and mobilization of the splenic flexure. Without an underlying pancreatic duct stricture, these fistulas will typically resolve with conservative management. However, if patients do go on to require surgery, then distal pancreatectomy is typically sufficient.

Pancreatic Fistula After Pancreatic Resection

Following pancreatic resection, a leak from either the divided edge of the pancreas or the pancreatic anastomosis is considered a postoperative pancreatic fistula. Rates of postoperative pancreatic fistula vary widely in series but approximate 20% for both distal pancreatectomy and pancreaticoduodenectomy and can have significant morbidity.[1,14,15] Numerous preoperative risk factors for pancreatic fistula have been identified, including male gender, jaundice, cardiovascular disease, operative time, intraoperative blood loss, type of pancreatico-digestive anastomosis, hospital volume, and the surgeon's experience.[16,17] Perhaps the most significant risk factors are pancreatic duct size and pancreatic texture. The management of a postoperative pancreatic fistula is generally supportive with drainage of any collections. Rarely are endoscopic or surgical therapies needed. To facilitate more accurate reporting of such fistulas, a uniform grading system has been developed (see **Table 1**).

Prevention of Fistula After Pancreatic Resection

Given the frequency of pancreatic fistulas following pancreatic resection, extensive research has looked at methods for prevention. In the setting of pancreaticoduodenectomy, the method of reconstruction (pancreaticojejunostomy vs pancreaticogastrostomy), the use of octreotide, the application of fibrin glue, and the type of anastomosis (invaginating, duct to mucosa, stented) have all been studied.[6,18–20]

Table 1
Grade of postoperative pancreatic fistula

Grade	A	B	C
Clinical conditions	Well	Often well	Ill appearing/bad
Specific treatment	No	Yes/no	Yes
US/CT (if obtained)	Negative	Negative/positive	Positive
Persistent drainage (after 3 wk)	No	Usually yes	Yes
Reoperation	No	No	Yes
Death related to fistula	No	No	Possibly yes
Signs of infections	No	Yes/no	Yes
Sepsis	No	No	Yes
Readmission	No	Yes/no	Yes/no

Drain output of any measurable volume of fluid on or after postoperative day 3 with an amylase content greater than 3 times the serum amylase activity.
Abbreviation: US, ultrasound.
Data from Bassi C, Dervenis C, Butturini G, et al. Postoperative pancreatic fistula: an international study group (ISGPF) definition. Surgery 2005;138(1):8–13.

No single method has been shown to be consistently better than the others. In the setting of distal pancreatectomy, numerous methods for transecting the pancreas and controlling the remnant have been investigated. They include stapled closure, sutured closure, transection and control with various energy devices, the application of fibrin glue, and coverage with autologous tissue.[21–23] The level of evidence varies dramatically among the studies; as in the case of pancreaticoduodenectomy, no method is reliably better than the others at lowering the fistula rate. Minimizing postoperative pancreatic fistulas remains a topic of intense investigation.

SUMMARY

The management of pancreatic fistulas can be complex and mandates a multidisciplinary approach. Basic principles of fistula control/patient stabilization, delineation of ductal anatomy, and definitive therapy remain of paramount importance.

REFERENCES

1. Bassi C, Dervenis C, Butturini G, et al. Postoperative pancreatic fistula: an international study group (ISGPF) definition. Surgery 2005;138(1):8–13.
2. Ho KM, Dobb GJ, Webb SA. A comparison of early gastric and post-pyloric feeding in critically ill patients: a meta-analysis. Intensive Care Med 2006;32(5): 639–49.
3. Andriulli A, Loperfido S, Napolitano G, et al. Incidence rates of post-ERCP complications: a systematic survey of prospective studies. Am J Gastroenterol 2007; 102(8):1781–8.
4. Fischer A, Benz S, Baier P, et al. Endoscopic management of pancreatic fistulas secondary to intraabdominal operation. Surg Endosc 2004;18(4):706–8.
5. Halttunen J, Weckman L, Kemppainen E, et al. The endoscopic management of pancreatic fistulas. Surg Endosc 2005;19(4):559–62.
6. Gans SL, van Westreenen HL, Kiewiet JJ, et al. Systematic review and meta-analysis of somatostatin analogues for the treatment of pancreatic fistula. Br J Surg 2012;99(6):754–60.
7. Cothren CC, McIntyre RC Jr, Johnson S, et al. Management of low-output pancreatic fistulas with fibrin glue. Am J Surg 2004;188(1):89–91.
8. Bakker OJ, van Baal MC, van Santvoort HC, et al. Endoscopic transpapillary stenting or conservative treatment for pancreatic fistulas in necrotizing pancreatitis: multicenter series and literature review. Ann Surg 2011;253(5):961–7.
9. Varadarajulu S, Noone TC, Tutuian R, et al. Predictors of outcome in pancreatic duct disruption managed by endoscopic transpapillary stent placement. Gastrointest Endosc 2005;61(4):568–75.
10. Nealon WH, Walser E. Duct drainage alone is sufficient in the operative management of pancreatic pseudocyst in patients with chronic pancreatitis. Ann Surg 2003;237(5):614–20 [discussion: 620–2].
11. Pearson EG, Scaife CL, Mulvihill SJ, et al. Roux-en-Y drainage of a pancreatic fistula for disconnected pancreatic duct syndrome after acute necrotizing pancreatitis. HPB (Oxford) 2012;14(1):26–31.
12. Pelaez-Luna M, Vege SS, Petersen BT, et al. Disconnected pancreatic duct syndrome in severe acute pancreatitis: clinical and imaging characteristics and outcomes in a cohort of 31 cases. Gastrointest Endosc 2008;68(1):91–7.
13. Irani S, Gluck M, Ross A, et al. Resolving external pancreatic fistulas in patients with disconnected pancreatic duct syndrome: using rendezvous techniques to avoid surgery (with video). Gastrointest Endosc 2012;76(3):586–593.e1–3.

14. Reeh M, Nentwich MF, Bogoevski D, et al. High surgical morbidity following distal pancreatectomy: still an unsolved problem. World J Surg 2011;35(5):1110–7.
15. Jensen EH, Portschy PR, Chowaniec J, et al. Meta-analysis of bioabsorbable staple line reinforcement and risk of fistula following pancreatic resection. J Gastrointest Surg 2013;17:267–72.
16. Ho V, Heslin MJ. Effect of hospital volume and experience on in-hospital mortality for pancreaticoduodenectomy. Ann Surg 2003;237(4):509–14.
17. Yang YM, Tian XD, Zhuang Y, et al. Risk factors of pancreatic leakage after pancreaticoduodenectomy. World J Gastroenterol 2005;11(16):2456–61.
18. Wente MN, Shrikhande SV, Muller MW, et al. Pancreaticojejunostomy versus pancreaticogastrostomy: systematic review and meta-analysis. Am J Surg 2007; 193(2):171–83.
19. Ochiai T, Sonoyama T, Soga K, et al. Application of polyethylene glycolic acid felt with fibrin sealant to prevent postoperative pancreatic fistula in pancreatic surgery. J Gastrointest Surg 2010;14(5):884–90.
20. Berger AC, Howard TJ, Kennedy EP, et al. Does type of pancreaticojejunostomy after pancreaticoduodenectomy decrease rate of pancreatic fistula? A randomized, prospective, dual institution trial. J Am Coll Surg 2009;208(5):738–47.
21. Diener MK, Seiler CM, Rossion I, et al. Efficacy of stapler versus hand-sewn closure after distal pancreatectomy (DISPACT): a randomised, controlled multicentre trial. Lancet 2011;377(9776):1514–22.
22. Zhou W, Lv R, Wang X, et al. Stapler vs suture closure of pancreatic remnant after distal pancreatectomy: a meta-analysis. Am J Surg 2010;200(4):529–36.
23. Carter TI, Fong ZV, Hyslop T, et al. A dual-institution randomized controlled trial of remnant closure after distal pancreatectomy: does the addition of a falciform patch and fibrin glue improve outcomes? J Gastrointest Surg 2013;17:102–9.

Type 2 Diabetes Mellitus and Pancreatic Cancer

John C. McAuliffe, MD, PhD, John D. Christein, MD*

KEYWORDS

- Pancreatic cancer • Type 2 diabetes mellitus • Pancreatectomy

KEY POINTS

- The cause of type 2 diabetes mellitus (DM2) in the context of pancreatic cancer (PC) is multifactorial.
- The pancreas is a complex organ orchestrating interrelated endocrine and exocrine pathways for normal absorption and metabolism of nutrients.
- DM2 may be a risk factor and harbinger of PC.
- DM2 increases the risk of pancreatic surgical intervention.
- Resection of the pancreas for cancer increases one's chance of DM2.

INTRODUCTION

Pancreatic cancer (PC) is the fourth leading cause of cancer-related mortality in the United States and up to 230,000 people worldwide will die of PC this year. Approximately 43,000 people will be diagnosed with PC in the United States this year.[1,2] With the rising incidence, it is unfortunate that the estimated overall 1-year survival is only 22% with less than 5% survival at 5 years. The only potentially curative modality is surgical resection; however, even with advances in cross-sectional imaging and endoscopic diagnostics, only 15% to 20% of patients will have resectable disease at presentation.[1] The median survival after complete resection can be up to 20 months with 5-year survival rates approaching 25%. Because the likelihood of a poor outcome for patients in all stages of PC, investigational options are used for all phases of disease management.[3]

The prognosis of PC is quite poor and the above figures underscore PC's aggressive nature and the need for early detection. Currently, there are no validated means of screening for PC. Patients presenting with symptoms of PC, which are usually vague and nonspecific, typically have complex comorbid conditions and age-associated factors, making operative treatment high-risk. Symptoms and signs, once present, often relate to advanced disease.

Department of Surgery, The Kirklin Clinic, UAB Medical Center, 1802 6th Avenue South, Birmingham, AL 35294, USA
* Corresponding author.
E-mail address: jchristein@uabmc.edu

Surg Clin N Am 93 (2013) 619–627
http://dx.doi.org/10.1016/j.suc.2013.02.003
0039-6109/13/$ – see front matter

Risk factors for PC are difficult to establish, but cigarette smoking, obesity, and type 2 diabetes mellitus (DM2) are factors that may be modified. DM2 affects up to 8% of the US population and is more commonly seen with increased age. Considering that DM2 is more common as age increases, much like PC, this association is often difficult to establish until other physical signs present. The relationship of PC and DM2 is complex and the mechanism is not fully understood. However, elucidating the interaction between PC and DM2 may lead to novel treatment strategies and establish a hope of early detection. Thus, for surgeons participating in the management of PC, the relationship of DM2 and PC, as well as the morbidity of DM2, in this patient population should be appreciated.

DIAGNOSIS OF DM2

Historically, DM2 was diagnosed based on fasting plasma glucose and oral glucose tolerance test values, and it was not until 1997 when these tests were validated with end-organ damage. In 1997, the Expert Committee on Diagnosis and Classification of Diabetes Mellitus sought to determine a threshold glucose level that caused end-organ damage, specifically retinopathy. From these studies, the diagnosis of DM2 was determined to be a fasting glucose of greater than or equal to 126 mg/dL and an oral glucose tolerance test of greater than or equal to 200 mg/dL.[4] Initially, glycosylated hemoglobin (HbA1c) was not included in the diagnostic criteria; however, now, with higher quality and standardized assays, its value is paramount. The diagnostic criteria for DM2 are summarized in **Table 1**.

ANATOMY AND PHYSIOLOGY OF ISLET CELLS

The pancreas consists of two main types of tissue, most of which is exocrine acinar cell mass. A much smaller percentage of the pancreatic mass is ellipsoid clusters of cells known as the pancreatic islets of Langerhans, the endocrine cells embedded in the exocrine tissue. Despite this, the islets receive 20% to 30% of the pancreatic blood flow, which is controlled by glucose levels, neural and hormonal pathways, and nitric oxide levels. A normal adult human pancreas may contain up to a million islets.

Each islet is a mass of polyhedral cells separated by fenestrated capillaries and a rich autonomic innervation. The islets are distributed throughout the pancreas but mostly concentrated to the tail. That being said, each islet's cellular composition differs for each segment of the pancreas, whereas β cells and Δ cells are evenly distributed throughout the pancreas. The pancreatic head and uncinate have a higher percentage of pancreatic polypeptide (PP) cells and few α cells, whereas the islets in the body and tail contain most of the α cells and few PP cells (**Table 2**).

Table 1 Diagnostic criteria for DM2		
Test	Cut-Off Value	Notes
Fasting plasma glucose	≥126 mg/dL	No caloric intake for 8 h
Glucose tolerance test	≥200 mg/dL	2 h after ingesting 75 g of glucose
HbA1c	≥6.5%	Must be National Glycohemoglobin Standardization Program-certified
Random plasma glucose	≥200 mg/dL	If patient has symptoms of hyperglycemic crisis

Table 2
Islet cells of the pancreas and function

Islet Cell	Pancreas Distribution	Hormone Secretion	Hormone Function
β	Evenly	Insulin	Glucose sequestration, glycogenesis, protein synthesis, fatty acid synthesis
α	Tail	Glucagon, ghrelin	Opposite of insulin
Δ	Evenly	Somatostatin	Decreased gastrointestinal exocrine and endocrine secretion
ε	Evenly	Ghrelin	Decreased insulin release and insulin action
PP	Head, uncinate	Pancreatic peptide	Decreased pancreatic exocrine and insulin secretion

In the islets, the α and β cells are the most numerous and secrete glucagon and insulin, respectively. The α cells tend to be concentrated at the periphery of islets, whereas β cells are more central, displaying the autocrine, paracrine, and hormonal functions of the individual islets. The other cells making up each islet are found in much smaller numbers and include Δ cells, ε cells, and PP cells, which secrete somatostatin, gastrin, ghrelin, and PP, respectively. In all, more than 20 different hormones have been identified to be secreted by the islets, making for a complex milieu of regulatory crossroads. The autonomic neurotransmitters acetylcholine (ACh) and noradrenaline affect islet cell secretion: ACh augments insulin and glucagon release, whereas noradrenaline inhibits glucose-induced insulin release and may also affect somatostatin and PP secretion.[5,6]

Insulin secretion is mediated by glucose, arginine, lysine, leucine, and free fatty acids circulating levels, as well as by the hormones glucagon and cholecystokinin.[7] Insulin secretion is inhibited by somatostatin, amylin, and hypoglycemia.[8] Insulin's function is to decrease serum glucose. To accomplish this task, it acts on various organs (particularly the liver) to reduce gluconeogenesis, glycogenolysis, fatty acid breakdown, and ketone formation while stimulating protein synthesis.

Glucagon, one of the counterregulatory hormones, initiates the opposite effects of insulin. It promotes hepatic glycogenolysis and gluconeogenesis, thus increasing serum glucose levels. Secretion of glucagon from α cells is inhibited by glucose and stimulated by arginine and alanine. Also, insulin and somatostatin inhibit glucagon secretion within the islet via a paracrine affect.

Somatostatin is a fundamental hormone regulating multiple processes in the body, including exocrine and endocrine function of the pancreas. Also, somatostatins modulate gastrointestinal and biliary motility, intestinal absorption, vascular tone, and cell proliferation.[9]

Collectively, hormones secreted by the islets orchestrate a complex physiologic balance controlling fuel storage and use.[10] Derangement of this balance perturbs glucose homeostasis and will lead to either hyperglycemia or hypoglycemia.[11]

DM2 is a heterogeneous disorder characterized by hyperglycemia. This hyperglycemia is related to a functional deficiency of insulin; specifically, decreased secretion from islets, decreased response to target organs, or increased counterregulatory hormones opposing insulin's action. Increased counterregulatory hormones, such as glucagon, will mimic the fasting state despite normal fuel homeostasis. The severity and clinical manifestations of DM2 is related to the functional ratios of the islet hormones.

RELATIONSHIP BETWEEN DM2 AND PC

Approximately 80% of patients with PC have frank DM2 or glucose intolerance.[12] The increased frequency of DM2 in patients with PC is well established but the question remains whether DM2 is due to PC from obstructive pancreatitis or a paracrine hormonal affect, or is it only a risk factor for PC.

In one study, 56% of patients with PC were diagnosed with DM2 concomitantly or within 2 years before the diagnosis of cancer. Although the association between the two diagnoses was significant, when controlling for duration of DM2, there was no longer a significant association. The investigators concluded that DM2 is not a risk factor for developing PC but acts more as a symptom of the tumor.[13]

In contrast, a meta-analysis shortly thereafter showed a relative risk of 2.0 for developing PC if a patient had DM2 for more than 5 years, touting DM2 as a risk factor for PC.[14] This study was updated in 2005 with increased follow-up, showing that individuals recently diagnosed with DM2 (<4 years) had a 50% greater risk of malignancy compared with those with DM2 for more than 5 years.[15] In general, risk assessment shows that DM2-associated PC was higher in newly-diagnosed patients compared with those with long-term DM2, alluding to the effects from the tumor. These studies suggest that new-onset DM2 may play a role in the early detection of PC, before the onset of classic symptoms such as jaundice, weight loss, and pain.

In another study from 2005, the association between new-onset DM2 and PC was demonstrated in that 1% of the newly diagnosed DM2 patients will be diagnosed with PC within 3 years.[16] Expanding on this theme, two studies in 2008 showed that DM2 was more prevalent and predominantly of new-onset among those with PC compared with controls.[17,18] These studies suggest that new-onset DM2 may be an early symptom for PC and a potential screening tool to better diagnose early, resectable PC.[19] Other studies go further to show that 71% of glucose intolerance found in PC patients is unknown before PC diagnosis, again suggesting that glucose intolerance or DM2 may be a consequence of PC and, therefore, an early sign of PC.[20,21]

The mechanism underlying the relationship of DM2 and PC is complex and likely includes metabolic, immunologic, and hormonal alterations intimately involved in tumorigenesis and tumor progression. As previously stated, DM2 is a consequence of a deficiency of functional insulin. This deficiency can be due to a lack of production or lack of end-organ response to insulin. In 2004, Chari and colleagues[22] showed that DM2 associated with PC is likely due to both decline in β-cell function and increased end-organ resistance. A subsequent meta-analysis indicated that elevated serum c-peptide to insulin ratio was associated with PC, implicating peripheral insulin resistance in the mechanism of DM2-associated PC.[23]

In response to insulin resistance, β-cell mass is increased with resultant hyperactivity due to hyperglycemia. Thus, the microenvironment of the pancreas is subjected to high local insulin levels such as those with insulin resistance or DM2. Evidence shows that insulin is mitogenic and augments cell proliferation and glucose use, one of the hallmarks of neoplasia. Also, as insulin increases so do the insulin-like growth factors, which are potent mediators of many tumor progression pathway models.[21,24–26] These data suggest that insulin resistance and DM2, through the direct action of insulin and its downstream signaling pathways, may potentiate and facilitate malignant transformation within the exocrine pancreas, thus leading to pancreatic ductal adenocarcinoma.

Moreover, PC cells also alter gene expression in skeletal muscles, a key end target of insulin's function. Basso and colleagues[27] showed that skeletal cell metabolism was dramatically altered following treatment with pancreatic cell line–conditioned media. During this therapy, myoblasts in culture had enhanced lactate production and proteolysis along with altered gene expression of tricarboxylic acid cycle mediators and glucose metabolism. This study strongly suggests that PC has endocrine function and may cause aberrant metabolism leading to DM2 in humans.

Therefore, the evidence shows that DM2 and PC are definitely interrelated. However, the inciting incident, PC versus DM2, remains unclear and of continued debate.[28] Further epidemiologic and basic science studies are required to mitigate confounding variables of an aged population and the pathologic hormonal milieu of DM2 and PC.[29,30]

Work-up for an Asymptomatic Patient with New-Onset DM2

Because evidence shows that DM2 and PC are interrelated, what should a clinician do for a patient presenting with new-onset DM2? Should an extensive workup ensue to evaluate for PC? As stated previously, most patients with PC are symptomatic (up to 70%),presenting with stage III or IV (unresectable) disease. The goal of screening patients is to diagnose a resectable PC and likely asymptomatic DM2. The American Diabetes Association (ADA) recommends DM2 screening for all individuals more than 45 years old every 3 years and screening individuals at an earlier age if they are over-weight (body mass index >25 kg/m^2) and have one additional risk factor for DM2. Risk factors for DM2 include obesity and family history, physical inactivity, non–white race, hypertension, hypercholesterolemia, polycystic ovarian disease, and cardiovascular disease. In 2010, the prevalence of DM2 in the United States was estimated to be 0.2% in individuals aged less than 20 years and 11.3% in individuals aged more than 20 years. In individuals aged more than 65 years, the prevalence of DM2 was 26.9% (ADA 2011). Therefore, most patients diagnosed with DM2 are in the same age group as those diagnosed with PC. Yet, most patients of this age have a risk factor for DM2, which has a substantially higher prevalence than PC. As such, there is no data or evidence to suggest that an asymptomatic patient with risk factors for DM2 presenting with new-onset DM2 should have a work-up for PC. However, for an asymptomatic patient without risk factors for DM2 presenting with new-onset DM2 may benefit from work up for PC or other causes of DM2. To the authors' knowledge, there is no evidence for this rare case, but we would suggest imaging of the pancreas by CT or endoscopic ultrasound (EUS) to begin a work-up for PC or other pancreatic disease leading to DM2. Evidence suggests that EUS is more accurate at diagnosing and staging small tumors (<3 cm) compared with CT.[31] Patients with PC less than 3 cm are likely asymptomatic. Thus, an asymptomatic patient with new onset DM2 without risk factors for DM2 may benefit from EUS to evaluate the pancreas for early, resectable, small lesions.

DM2 AND RESECTION OF PC

Systems improvements have, to date, successfully improved the quality of patient care in the perioperative period following major pancreatic resections. Recent data suggest that various prognostic factors influence surgical outcomes. These prognostic factors are in the process of validation through high-volume ongoing work on a multi-institutional scale. Numerous risk scoring systems based on these identified risk factors have been devised with the aim of delineating those patients most suitable for surgical intervention.[32–40] PC, with its myriad of comorbid burdens, provides a setting to apply these risk predicting tools. Moreover, achievement of benchmark outcomes is especially important in the setting of PC, in light of few resections for cure with a narrow margin for operative success and rare long-term survival.

The impact of DM2 on surgical outcomes is well documented. Two studies by Chagpar and colleagues[41] and Chu and colleagues[42] show that preoperative DM2 increases operative complications following pancreatic surgery.

In the Chagpar and colleagues[41] study, 518 patients underwent resection for PC, of which 13% were treated with insulin before resection. In univariate analysis, insulin-dependent DM2 increased the 90-day mortality following resection from 4.8% to 13% (P-value = .02). After multivariate analysis, insulin usage predicted early mortality with an odds ratio of 3.0 following pancreatic resection. The impact of DM2 on operative mortality following pancreatectomy was only seen in the insulin-dependent group, and directed counseling of these patients is warranted.

Chu and colleagues[42] described 251 patients undergoing resection for PC, in which 46% had preoperative DM2. When controlling for age, body mass index, albumin levels, operation type, operative time, and pancreatic firmness, preoperative DM2 independently predicted postoperative pancreatic fistula, through multivariate analysis, with an odds ratio of 4.3.

Although DM2 does adversely affect operative morbidity and mortality, DM2 also affects long-term survival for patients with PC. In 2010, Chu and colleagues[43] presented a series of 209 patients undergoing resection for PC, in which 45% had either long-standing or new-onset DM2. Patients with DM2 had larger tumors (>3 cm) and DM2 was independently associated with reduced median survival (15 vs 17 months, P = .02, hazard ratio 1.55) when controlling for age, comorbidities, and tumor size. Not only was survival decreased, this association seemed to be more pronounced for patients with new-onset DM2.

With the mounting evidence that DM2 portends decreased survival in patients undergoing resection for PC, Hartwig and colleagues[44] reviewed 1071 patients undergoing resection for PC to determine positive and negative prognostic factors of long-term survival and to improve on the American Joint Committee on Cancer (AJCC) staging system. In multivariate analysis, insulin-dependent DM2 was independently associated with poor prognosis and decreased survival. Following this, in 2012, Cannon and colleagues[45] confirmed the above results and showed that preoperative DM2 decreased both disease-free and overall survival for patients undergoing resection for PC.

Following resection for PC, many patients have been shown to have altered glucose metabolism. Interestingly, some studies describe increased endocrine insufficiency, whereas others show that improvement may be seen in some patients.[46–49] Resection not only removes functioning islets but also removes the potentially diabetogenic PC. Predicting the outcome of glycemic control in a particular patient undergoing resection for PC is difficult and, to date, cannot be done. However, White and colleagues[50] evaluated 101 patients undergoing pancreatectomy for PC in which 41% had preoperative DM2. After resection, 20% developed DM2, whereas 35% of patients with preoperative DM2 showed improvement in control or cure of their DM2. There is definitely conflicting evidence in the literature but it seems clear that, in some patients, the pancreatic adenocarcinoma is diabetogenic.

SUMMARY

As the operative morbidity and mortality of pancreatectomy at high-volume centers has improved, incidence has increased and survival has remained mostly unchanged. PC symptoms are continuing to present late in the course of disease and most patients are not surgical candidates when discovered. In light of recent observational and basic science reports, tumorigenesis of PC and the pathophysiology of DM2 emerge as intertwined pathways. The cause of each disease entity has been discussed and seems to be linked in a subset of patients who develop PC. Paramount to this discussion, however, is the hope of better understanding that the diagnosis of DM2 suggests pancreatic dysfunction and possible early carcinogenesis. Additionally, DM2 is a significant comorbidity predicting worse outcomes in patients undergoing pancreatic resection as part of the treatment of PC. Better understanding of PC and metabolic derangements such as DM2 will translate to improved morbidity and mortality for patients accursed with PC.

REFERENCES

1. Sharma C, Eltawil KM, Renfrew PD, et al. Advances in diagnosis, treatment and palliation of pancreatic carcinoma: 1990-2010. World J Gastroenterol 2011;17(7): 867–97.
2. Vincent A, Herman J, Schulick R, et al. Pancreatic cancer. Lancet 2011; 378(9791):607–20.
3. Panel NP. Pancreatic adenocarcinoma. National Comprehensive Cancer Network Clinical Practice Guidelines in Oncology 2012.
4. American Diabetes Association. Executive summary: Standards of medical care in diabetes—2012. Diabetes Care 2012;35(Suppl 1):S4–10.
5. Kleinman RM, Gingerich R, Ohning G, et al. Intraislet regulation of pancreatic polypeptide secretion in the isolated perfused rat pancreas. Pancreas 1997; 15(4):384–91.
6. Brunicardi FC, Druck P, Seymour NE, et al. Splanchnic neural regulation of pancreatic polypeptide release in the isolated perfused human pancreas. Am J Surg 1989;157(1):50–7.
7. Ebert R, Creutzfeldt W. Gastrointestinal peptides and insulin secretion. Diabetes Metab Rev 1987;3(1):1–26.
8. Kleinman R, Gingerich R, Ohning G, et al. The influence of somatostatin on glucagon and pancreatic polypeptide secretion in the isolated perfused human pancreas. Int J Pancreatol 1995;18(1):51–7.
9. Yamada Y, Post SR, Wang K, et al. Cloning and functional characterization of a family of human and mouse somatostatin receptors expressed in brain, gastrointestinal tract, and kidney. Proc Natl Acad Sci U S A 1992;89(1): 251–5.
10. Gerich JE, Campbell PJ, Kennedy FP. Non-beta-cell islet abnormalities in noninsulin-dependent diabetes mellitus. Prog Clin Biol Res 1988;265:133–50.
11. Cryer PE. Minireview: glucagon in the pathogenesis of hypoglycemia and hyperglycemia in diabetes. Endocrinology 2012;153(3):1039–48.
12. Permert J, Ihse I, Jorfeldt L, et al. Pancreatic cancer is associated with impaired glucose metabolism. Eur J Surg 1993;159(2):101–7.
13. Gullo L, Pezzilli R, Morselli-Labate AM, et al. Diabetes and the risk of pancreatic cancer. N Engl J Med 1994;331(2):81–4.
14. Everhart J, Wright D. Diabetes mellitus as a risk factor for pancreatic cancer. A meta-analysis. JAMA 1995;273(20):1605–9.
15. Huxley R, Ansary-Moghaddam A, Berrington de González A, et al. Type-II diabetes and pancreatic cancer: a meta-analysis of 36 studies. Br J Cancer 2005; 92(11):2076–83.
16. Chari ST, Leibson CL, Rabe KG, et al. Probability of pancreatic cancer following diabetes: a population-based study. Gastroenterology 2005;129(2): 504–11.

17. Pannala R, Leirness JB, Bamlet WR, et al. Prevalence and clinical profile of pancreatic cancer-associated diabetes mellitus. Gastroenterology 2008;134(4): 981–7.

18. Chari ST, Leibson CL, Rabe KG, et al. Pancreatic cancer-associated diabetes mellitus: prevalence and temporal association with diagnosis of cancer. Gastroenterology 2008;134(1):95–101.

19. Pannala R, Basu A, Petersen GM, et al. New-onset diabetes: a potential clue to the early diagnosis of pancreatic cancer. Lancet Oncol 2009;10(1):88–95.

20. Schwarts SS, Zeidler A, Moossa AR, et al. A prospective study of glucose tolerance, insulin, C-peptide, and glucagon responses in patients with pancreatic carcinoma. Am J Dig Dis 1978;23(12):1107–14.

21. Li D. Diabetes and pancreatic cancer. Mol Carcinog 2012;51(1):64–74.

22. Chari ST, Zapiach M, Yadav D, et al. Beta-cell function and insulin resistance evaluated by HOMA in pancreatic cancer subjects with varying degrees of glucose intolerance. Pancreatology 2005;5(2–3):229–33.

23. Pisani P. Hyper-insulinaemia and cancer, meta-analyses of epidemiological studies. Arch Physiol Biochem 2008;114(1):63–70.

24. Powell DR, Suwanichkul A, Cubbage ML, et al. Insulin inhibits transcription of the human gene for insulin-like growth factor-binding protein-1. J Biol Chem 1991; 266(28):18868–76.

25. Stoeltzing O, Liu W, Reinmuth N, et al. Regulation of hypoxia-inducible factor-1alpha, vascular endothelial growth factor, and angiogenesis by an insulin-like growth factor-I receptor autocrine loop in human pancreatic cancer. Am J Pathol 2003;163(3):1001–11.

26. Ohmura E, Okada M, Onoda N, et al. Insulin-like growth factor I and transforming growth factor alpha as autocrine growth factors in human pancreatic cancer cell growth. Cancer Res 1990;50(1):103–7.

27. Basso D, Millino C, Greco E, et al. Altered glucose metabolism and proteolysis in pancreatic cancer cell conditioned myoblasts: searching for a gene expression pattern with a microarray analysis of 5000 skeletal muscle genes. Gut 2004; 53(8):1159–66.

28. Magruder JT, Elahi D, Andersen DK. Diabetes and pancreatic cancer: chicken or egg? Pancreas 2011;40(3):339–51.

29. Pezzilli R, Casadei R, Morselli-Labate AM. Is type 2 diabetes a risk factor for pancreatic cancer? JOP 2009;10(6):705–6.

30. Li D, Yeung SC, Hassan MM, et al. Antidiabetic therapies affect risk of pancreatic cancer. Gastroenterology 2009;137(2):482–8.

31. Varadarajulu S, Eloubeidi MA. The role of endoscopic ultrasonography in the evaluation of pancreatico-biliary cancer. Surg Clin North Am 2010;90(2): 251–63.

32. Hutter MM, Rowell KS, Devaney LA, et al. Identification of surgical complications and deaths: an assessment of the traditional surgical morbidity and mortality conference compared with the American College of Surgeons-National Surgical Quality Improvement Program. J Am Coll Surg 2006;203(5):618–24.

33. Kelly KJ, Greenblatt DY, Wan Y, et al. Risk stratification for distal pancreatectomy utilizing ACS-NSQIP: preoperative factors predict morbidity and mortality. J Gastrointest Surg 2011;15(2):250–9 [discussion: 259–61].

34. Parikh P, Shiloach M, Cohen ME, et al. Pancreatectomy risk calculator: an ACS-NSQIP resource. HPB (Oxford) 2010;12(7):488–97.

35. Pitt HA, Kilbane M, Strasberg SM, et al. ACS-NSQIP has the potential to create an HPB-NSQIP option. HPB (Oxford) 2009;11(5):405–13.

36. Pratt W, Joseph S, Callery MP, et al. POSSUM accurately predicts morbidity for pancreatic resection. Surgery 2008;143(1):8–19.
37. Charlson ME, Sax FL, MacKenzie CR, et al. Resuscitation: how do we decide? A prospective study of physicians' preferences and the clinical course of hospitalized patients. JAMA 1986;255(10):1316–22.
38. Hill JS, Zhou Z, Simons JP, et al. A simple risk score to predict in-hospital mortality after pancreatic resection for cancer. Ann Surg Oncol 2010;17(7):1802–7.
39. Venkat R, Puhan MA, Schulick RD, et al. Predicting the risk of perioperative mortality in patients undergoing pancreaticoduodenectomy: a novel scoring system. Arch Surg 2011;146(11):1277–84.
40. Vollmer CM, Sanchez N, Gondek S, et al. A root-cause analysis of mortality following major pancreatectomy. J Gastrointest Surg 2012;16(1):89–102 [discussion: 102–3].
41. Chagpar RB, Martin RC, Ahmad SA, et al. Medically managed hypercholesterolemia and insulin-dependent diabetes mellitus preoperatively predicts poor survival after surgery for pancreatic cancer. J Gastrointest Surg 2011;15(4):551–7.
42. Chu CK, Mazo AE, Sarmiento JM, et al. Impact of diabetes mellitus on perioperative outcomes after resection for pancreatic adenocarcinoma. J Am Coll Surg 2010;210(4):463–73.
43. Chu CK, Mazo AE, Goodman M, et al. Preoperative diabetes mellitus and long-term survival after resection of pancreatic adenocarcinoma. Ann Surg Oncol 2010;17(2):502–13.
44. Hartwig W, Hackert T, Hinz U, et al. Pancreatic cancer surgery in the new millennium: better prediction of outcome. Ann Surg 2011;254(2):311–9.
45. Cannon RM, LeGrand R, Chagpar RB, et al. Multi-institutional analysis of pancreatic adenocarcinoma demonstrating the effect of diabetes status on survival after resection. HPB (Oxford) 2012;14(4):228–35.
46. Pfeffer F, Nauck MA, Benz S, et al. Secondary diabetes in pancreatic carcinoma and after pancreatectomy: pathophysiology, therapeutic peculiarities and prognosis. Z Gastroenterol 1999;(Suppl 1):10–4 [in German].
47. Hamilton L, Jeyarajah DR. Hemoglobin A1c can be helpful in predicting progression to diabetes after Whipple procedure. HPB (Oxford) 2007;9(1):26–8.
48. Permert J, Ihse I, Jorfeldt L, et al. Improved glucose metabolism after subtotal pancreatectomy for pancreatic cancer. Br J Surg 1993;80(8):1047–50.
49. Litwin J, Dobrowolski S, Orłowska-Kunikowska E, et al. Changes in glucose metabolism after Kausch-Whipple pancreatectomy in pancreatic cancer and chronic pancreatitis patients. Pancreas 2008;36(1):26–30.
50. White MA, Agle SC, Fuhr HM, et al. Impact of pancreatic cancer and subsequent resection on glycemic control in diabetic and nondiabetic patients. Am Surg 2011;77(8):1032–7.

Screening and Surgical Outcomes of Familial Pancreatic Cancer

Adam W. Templeton, MD*, Teresa A. Brentnall, MD

KEYWORDS

- Familial pancreatic cancer • Peutz-Jeghers syndrome
- Pancreatic intraepithelial neoplasia • Intraductal papillary mucinous neoplasm
- Mucinous cystic neoplasm

KEY POINTS

- Ten percent of pancreatic cancers have familial inheritance; most of the susceptibility genes for familial pancreatic cancer (FPC) have yet to be determined.
- Utility analysis suggests that pancreatic cancer screening is most cost-effective in individuals whose lifetime risk of pancreatic cancer is 16% or greater.
- Intraductal papillary mucinous neoplasm and pancreatic intraepithelial neoplasia are precursor lesions for FPC; these lesions are higher grade, more common, and multifocal in individuals with FPC compared with patients with sporadic adenocarcinoma and are rarely found in individuals with no history of pancreatic disease.
- High-risk individuals for pancreatic cancer can have abnormal findings on endoscopic ultrasound and magnetic resonance imaging/magnetic resonance cholangiopancreatography including cysts, chronic inflammatory changes, and solid lesions.
- Screening of high-risk individuals, combined with appropriate surgical management, can detect and remove precursor lesions and early pancreatic adenocarcinoma.

INTRODUCTION

Pancreatic cancer remains a lethal disease. In the United States there were 43,920 estimated new cases of pancreatic cancer and almost as many deaths (37,390) in 2012. Although pancreatic cancer accounts for only a small percentage of cancer cases diagnosed in the US, it is the fourth leading cause of cancer death. Unlike breast, colorectal, and prostate cancer, death rates have not declined appreciably in the last 20 years despite advancements in chemotherapy, diagnostic imaging,

Funding Sources: Nil.
Conflict of Interest: Nil.
Department of Gastroenterology, Digestive Diseases Center, University of Washington, Box Number 356424, 1959 Northeast Pacific Street, Seattle, WA 98195, USA
* Corresponding author.
E-mail address: templeaw@uw.edu

and the understanding of genetic risk factors. Pancreatic cancer, like ovarian cancer, continues to be diagnosed late in progression, often with metastatic disease. Five-year survival correspondingly remains low at only 5%.[1] Early detection of stage 1 disease with curative resection can improve 5-year survival rates upwards of 60%.[2,3] However, detection of asymptomatic early stage disease in the general population has remained elusive.

Although it remains cost-prohibitive to screen the general population for pancreatic cancer, models show that screening of high-risk individuals less than the age of 70 years and who have a lifetime risk of pancreatic cancer greater than or equal to 16% is cost-effective.[4] Approximately 10% of pancreatic cancer is estimated to have familial inheritance.[5,6] Depending on the penetrance of the gene, the risk of cancer in any one individual in these families developing pancreatic cancer can be upwards of 38% by age 70 years.[7] As such, several centers have implemented screening programs for individuals at high risk for developing pancreatic cancer and offer surgical management for concerning precursor findings.

Familial Pancreatic Cancer

Formally defined, familial pancreatic cancer (FPC) is a heterogenous syndrome characterized by a family with 2 or more first-degree relatives with pancreatic cancer, not associated with another described familial hereditary cancer syndrome. Extensive study of familial pancreatic kindreds is ongoing with national and international tumor registries including the North American National Familial Pancreatic Tumor Registry (NFPTR), the German National Case Collection of Familial Pancreatic Cancer (FaPaCa), and the European Registry of Hereditary Pancreatitis and Familial Pancreatic Cancer (EUROPAC).[8–10] Klein and colleagues[7] performed the largest prospective analysis of 5179 individuals from 838 kindreds with FPC. Patients with a single first-degree relative (FDR) affected with pancreatic cancer had a 4.5-fold increased risk of developing pancreatic cancer, 2 FDRs increased the risk to 6.4-fold, and 3 FDRs increased the risk to 32-fold. These numbers have held true in other population analyses.[9,11]

Modeling suggests that unidentified genetic factor(s) drive this familial clustering.[12] At least in European registries, 50% to 80% of families have a pattern of autosomal dominant inheritance.[9,10] Genome-wide association studies suggest susceptibility loci of sporadic pancreatic cancer located at 1p32, 5p15, and 13q22.[13] Large genomic studies are underway to identify the main genetic causes of FPC. An inherited mutation in the highly conserved region of 90-kD palladin (PALLD), an embryonic protein involved in cell motility and invasion, led to highly penetrant FPC associated with prodromal diabetes in one family.[14] To date, this is the only gene indentified in a family with FPC.

Anticipation, the phenomenon whereby successive generations develop the disease at an earlier age than the parent generation, has been shown to affect ~60% to 85% of FPC families in some registries.[8,15] Age of onset in a family member does not seem to affect risk in sporadic pancreatic cancer; however, an early age of onset in an FPC family member (age 40 years) has a marked increase in cumulative risk (19.2%–40%).[16]

Extrapancreatic malignancies are associated with FPC, and it has been hypothesized that there are pure pancreatic cancer families without associated tumors and families with associated tumors. In a Swedish registry, pancreatic cancer was associated with lung, rectal, and endometrial cancer, and melanoma.[17] A German study of 94 histologically confirmed FPC families had increased incidence of breast, colon, and lung cancer.[8] The NFPTR reported an increased risk of death from breast, ovarian, colon, and bile duct cancer.[18]

Known Genetic Syndromes with Increased Risk of Pancreatic Cancer

At present, approximately 20% of FPC can be attributed to a known genetic syndrome.[5] These syndromes are grouped into hereditary cancer syndromes and syndromes associated with chronic inflammation of the pancreas. The most common identified heritable pancreatic cancer syndromes include Peutz-Jeghers syndrome, familial atypical multiple mole melanoma (FAMMM), hereditary breast-ovarian cancer (HBOC; including BRCA1 and BRCA2), hereditary nonpolyposis colorectal carcinoma (HNPCC), and familial adenomatous polyposis (FAP). These syndromes have considerable heterogeneity in their relative risk of developing pancreatic cancer (Table 1); individuals with known FAP, BRCA1, or BRCA2 have approximately a 5% lifetime risk of pancreatic cancer, whereas the lifetime risk in Peutz-Jeghers is as great as 36%.[19,20] The number of affected FDRs and environmental factors can further mitigate this genetic predisposition. Syndromes that lead to an increased risk of pancreatic cancer caused by chronic inflammation of the pancreas are hereditary pancreatitis and, to a lesser extent, cystic fibrosis.

Table 1
Syndromes associated with FPC

	Relative Risk of Pancreatic Cancer	Cumulative Lifetime Risk by Age 70 y (%)	Gene(s) Identified	Extrapancreatic Malignancy
FPC				
1 FDR with PC	2-fold to 3-fold	—	Linkage 1p32, 5p15,	Lung, colon, breast
2 FDRs with PC	6-fold	~40	and 13q22,	
≥3 FDRs with PC	14–32-fold	—	PALLD[a]	
Hereditary Cancer Syndrome				
FAP	2-fold to 3-fold	5	APC	Colon, duodenum, stomach
Hereditary Breast Ovarian Cancer	3.5-fold to 10-fold	5	BRCA1 BRCA2 PALB2	Breast, ovarian, prostate
Lynch syndrome (HNPCC)	8.6-fold	<5	MLH1, MLH2, MSH6	Uterine, bladder, skin, ovary, bile duct, kidney, ureter
FAMMM	13-fold to 47-fold	17	P16/ CDKN2A	Melanoma
Peutz-Jeghers	132-fold	36	STK11	Breast, small intestine, lung, esophagus, stomach, uterus, ovary
Syndromes of Chronic Inflammation				
Hereditary pancreatitis	50-fold to 80-fold	40	PRSS1, SPINK1	—
Cystic fibrosis	5-fold	<5	CFTR	Bile duct cancer

Abbreviation: PC, pancreatic cancer.
[a] PALLD mutation is rare and has only been identified in 1 FPC family.

The remaining 80% of cases with an inherited predisposition are covered by the term FPC, and the susceptibility genes have yet to be identified.[21]

Other Risk Factors

A nested case-control study of factors that affect tumorigenesis in FPC included 251 members of 28 families with 2 or more members with pancreatic cancer (**Table 2**).[22] Smoking was an independent risk factor (odds ratio [OR] 3.7; 95% confidence interval [CI] 1.8–7.6), with FPC smokers developing cancer 1 decade earlier than FPC non-smokers (59 vs 69 years of age; P = .01). Nitrosamine tobacco metabolites have been found in the pancreatic juice of smokers compared with nonsmokers.[23] The number of affected FDRs also increased risk for development of pancreatic cancer in any given kindred (OR 1.4 more than the baseline risk per each additional affected family member; 95% CI 1.1–1.9). In addition, adult-onset diabetes is a risk factor for pancreatic neoplastic progression including development of pancreatic intraepithelial neoplasia (PanIN) 2/3, intraductal papillary mucinous neoplasm (IPMN), and cancer in FPC kindreds (OR 5.8; 95% CI 1.3–25.2). These environmental and clinical findings parallel the risk factor data from sporadic pancreatic cancer[24,25] and can be taken into account when determining who to put into screening and when to start screening (see **Table 2**). Risk stratification can ensure that the individuals at highest risk undergo cost-effective screening. PancPRO is a free risk assessment tool that can aid in screening decision making for management of individuals with FPC.[26]

PATHOPHYSIOLOGY

Pancreatic cancer arises from 3 precursor lesions: PanIN, IPMN, and mucinous cystic neoplasm (MCN). PanIN and IPMN are thought to be the primary source of malignancy in FPC.[6] This article does not further address MCN. Both PanIN and IPMN have separate characteristic genetic changes underlying progression and risk for eventual conversion to invasive adenocarcinoma.

PanIN

Of the precursor lesions, PanINs are the most commonly found lesions[27] and are defined as microscopic flat or papillary, noninvasive epithelial neoplasms arising in pancreatic ducts.[28] The neoplastic path from PanIN to malignancy follows a progression of normal microscopic epithelium to hyperplasia (PanIN-1), to low-grade dysplasia (PanIN-2), to high-grade dysplasia/carcinoma in situ (PanIN-3), before developing into invasive adenocarcinoma (**Fig. 1**). The genetic events that correlate

Table 2
Conditional logistic regression analysis of factors associated with pancreatic cancer risk among members of FPC kindreds

Factor	PC Cases Only OR[a] (95% CI)	PC or PanIN/IPMN Cases OR[a] (95% CI)
Ever smoking	3.7 (1.8–7.6)	4.1 (2.0–8.2)
No. of affected FDR	1.4 (1.1–1.9) per affected FDR	1.4 (1.1–2.0) per affected FDR
History of diabetes	2.1 (0.4–10.9)	5.8 (1.3–25.2)
Male gender	1.0 (05–2.1)	0.9 (0.5–1.9)

Abbreviation: CI, confidence interval.
  [a] Individual ORs adjusted for each of the other variables in the table and for age, number of affected second-degree relatives, prior diagnosis of nonpancreatic cancer, and relationship to other affected relatives (parent vs sibling).

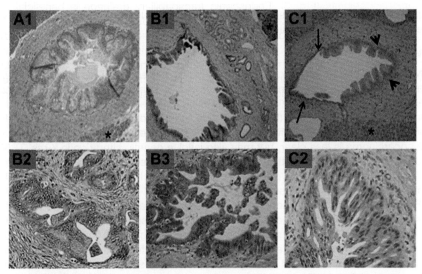

Fig. 1. PanIN lesions noted in pancreata of 3 different individuals with FPC (*A–C*) show the multifocality of the disease and the range of neoplastic progression that can be present within a single pancreas. PanIN-1 and 2 are noted in *A1*, *B1*, and *C1*, whereas PanIN-3 is present in *B2*, *B3*, and *C2*. (*C1*) Note the normal-appearing epithelial cells (*arrows*) adjacent to PanIN2 cells (*arrowheads*) within the same duct. Normal epithelial cells are cuboid and uniform in size and shape. In contrast, the cells in PanIN2 are elongated with enlarged atypical nuclei. (*B2*, *B3*, *C2*) Note the lush papillary projections of atypical cells filling the ductal lumen in the PanIN-3 lesions. Some of the pleomorphic nuclei have lost polarity and are no longer oriented to the basement membrane. Asterisks denote the normal-appearing acinar cells adjacent to PanIN lesions in some pancreata.

with this progression include telomere shortening and activating mutations in the k-ras oncogene (PanIN-1), inactivation of the tumor suppressor gene CDKN2A (PanIN-2), and then genetic inactivation of the cell regulator TP53, SMAD4 (transforming growth factor beta), and/or the tumor suppressor gene BRCA2 (PanIN-3).[29,30] Recent studies reveal that the genetic events, such as k-ras mutation, TP53 inactivation, and RNA expression changes are similar in sporadic pancreatic cancer compared with FPC neoplastic progression.[31,32]

The prevalence of PanIN lesions increases with age and they are more common in patients with chronic pancreatitis or adenocarcinoma than in individuals who have no history of pancreatic disease.[33,34] In a study by Andea and colleagues,[33] pancreata resected for adenocarcinoma were compared with pancreata resected for other reasons (trauma, metastatic disease to the pancreas, chronic pancreatitis). Only 16% of control pancreata had PanIN lesions, all of which were low-grade PanIN-1 and PanIN-2. In contrast, 82% of pancreata with adenocarcinoma had concomitant PanIN and 40% of these lesions were PanIN-3.[35,36] The timeline for progression of PanIN to metastatic disease is unclear. Rough estimates suggest a 1% probability of a single PanIN lesion progressing to invasive cancer.[37] Because PanIN lesions are multifocal throughout the pancreas of affected individuals with FPC, the risk of progression could be substantial. In hereditary nonpolyposis colon cancer, another familial cancer syndrome, it is known that leaving in place even a small precursor lesion, such as a colonic adenoma, provides a high likelihood of progression to cancer. Apart from increased initiation of precursor lesions, there is an 8-fold increased rate for the progression of precancerous lesions into cancer.[38]

IPMN

IPMN are defined as grossly visible mucin-producing epithelial neoplasms ($\geq$1 cm) that arise within the main pancreatic duct or one of its branches.[28] IPMN are further classified as incipient IPMN (<1 cm with IPMN characteristics), mild dysplasia (adenoma), moderate dysplasia (borderline), and marked dysplasia (carcinoma in situ) before progression to invasive carcinoma.[39] The genetic progression of IPMN to adenocarcinoma is less clear, but may also involve genetic alteration in k-ras, TP53, MUC, and SMAD4.[40,41] Activation of GNAS (G protein mediated signaling) and RNF43 (ubiquitin-dependent protein degradation), which have not been seen in the smaller PanIN lesions, are also implicated.[29]

By their size, IPMN are macroscopically more visible and characteristics on noninvasive imaging can help delineate risk for malignancy in sporadic disease. With regard to sporadic IPMN, involvement with the main pancreatic duct (MD), as opposed to a side branch; pancreatic ductal dilatation; as well as features such as mural nodules, advanced size, and malignant cytologic lesions all suggest higher potential for invasive malignancy.[42] As with PanIN lesions, the timeline to progression is not clear. In a review of all patients undergoing sporadic IPMN resection at a single tertiary center, Sohn and colleagues[39] speculated that, based on age at resection, there seemed to be a 5-year lag time from IPMN to invasive cancer. Asymptomatic side-branch IPMN is generally thought to be low risk for neoplastic progression in the sporadic setting. In the familial setting, this may not necessarily hold true. Familial IPMN has been described and, as with FPC precursor PanIN lesions, the genetic causes have yet to be determined.[43] With regard to neoplastic risk of IPMN in the familial setting, concurrent pancreatic ductal adenocarcinoma is more common in IPMN patients with a family history of pancreatic cancer compared with those without a family history (11.1% vs 2.9%, $P = .02$).[44,45] Whether time to progression of IPMN would be accelerated in the familial setting is unknown. In addition, IPMN seems to be associated with increased risk of extrapancreatic malignancy.[46]

Extent and Grade of Precursor Lesions in FPC

Consecutive autopsy studies of patients with no previous history of pancreatic cancer revealed that PanIN-1 is common, PanIN-2 is uncommon, and PanIN-3 is extremely rare in the general population.[47,48] In contrast, both IPMN and PanIN are found with greater frequency and at higher grade in patients with FPC compared with controls.[35,36,44] In particular, high-grade precursor lesions in FPC pancreata are notable for their panorgan multifocality.[44,49] In a comparison study of 51 resected pancreatic tissues from patients with a strong family history of pancreatic cancer versus pancreatic tissue from patients with sporadic pancreatic cancer, Shi and colleagues[35] found a 2.75-fold increased relative rate of PanIN per square centimeter, and an increase in the number of PanIN-3 lesions. High-grade incipient IPMN were only found in familial cases and not in the sporadic cases.

Extrapancreatic rests can undergo malignant degeneration in tandem with the main organ in individuals with FPC and should be sought out if an individual undergoes pancreatic surgery.[50] Observational studies of patients with FPC in screening programs suggest that the changes documented by imaging (ie, going from normal magnetic resonance imaging [MRI]/magnetic resonance cholangiopancreatography [MRCP] or endoscopic ultrasound [EUS] to metastatic disease) can occur over the course of 1 to 2 years in some cases and over a period of a decade or more in others

(Brentnall, unpublished data).[51] Natural history data of sporadic patients with retained PanIN lesions in the pancreatic remnant after partial surgical resection supports this variation in time to cancer progression.[52]

PANCREATIC CANCER SCREENING

Mortality in pancreatic cancer is driven largely by late diagnosis; however, if malignancy can be caught early, when tumors are less than 1 cm and without nodal involvement, 5-year prognosis can improve from 5% to 60%.[2] As such, once high-risk groups are identified, specialty centers have begun exploring screening programs for pancreatic cancer. To date, screening has been well tolerated[53–55] and, at least in 1 study, patients have had decreased cancer-related thoughts, cancer-related avoidant thoughts, and cancer worry.[53] However, screening programs have used heterogeneous approaches in the type and age of patients screened, imaging used, and definitions of clinical success. Despite these variable approaches, there has been some success in the detection of early cancers and high-grade IPMN/PanIN-3.

Who Should Be Screened?

Since an initial international consensus conference in 2003, general expert agreement exists that high-risk individuals with at least 5% to 10% relative risk of developing pancreatic cancer (see **Table 1**), and who would be suitable candidates for pancreatic surgery, should undergo screening at specialty centers.[21] A subsequent utility analysis suggested that high-risk individuals with a lifetime pancreatic cancer risk of 16% or greater provide the most cost-effective cohort for screening.[4]

Initial suggestions recommended starting screening at age 40 years or 10 years before the youngest age of onset in a family member. This recommendation is based largely on the following: (1) Klein and colleagues'[7] 2004 cohort study in which the youngest identified individual was 45 years of age and the age group with highest risk was between 45 and 65 years of age[7]; (2) the knowledge that, in some centers, FPC shows anticipation[56]; and (3) experience with colorectal cancer screening.[57] However, this may not be a cost-effective approach because of the paucity of high-risk individuals who get cancer or high-grade lesions before the age of 50 years. More recently, Ludwig and colleagues[49] reported the greatest yield in a screening program using MRCP followed by EUS. Abnormalities were most prevalent in patients more than 65 years of age (35% of patients >65 years) compared with 3% of those age 55 to 65 years and 3% of patients younger than age 55 years. The youngest patient in this series to have a high-risk lesion (PanIN-3, high-grade IPMN) or cancer was a 58 year-old man with T3N0 pancreatic adenocarcinoma. Overall, the prevalence of high-grade neoplasia or cancer in patients younger than 50 years varies in published literature; however, when neoplasia does occur in young individuals (<age 50 years) it usually does so in the setting in which other family members from that kindred have had early onset of cancer as well.[44,57,58] In sum, it may be most cost-effective to start screening in high-risk individuals at age 50 years or 10 years before the earliest age of pancreatic cancer onset in the family. Mitigating factors that could additionally affect the timing for commencement of screening include smoking, and new-onset diabetes; patients who are symptomatic should also be considered when deciding when to start screening (**Table 3**).

A separate issue is when to stop screening in high-risk individuals. As individuals age they have competing causes of death. Common sense dictates that screening is likely not productive for patients who are in poor health or who are poor operative

Table 3
Factors that influence selection of high-risk individuals for pancreatic cancer screening

	Genetic Predisposition	Environmental	Family History	Symptomatic
Surveillance if any one factor is present	Peutz-Jegher, P16 gene (FAMM), palladin	—	2 or more family members, one of whom is a FDR	—
Surveillance considered if a genetic predisposition is present (column 1) combined with other factors	BRCA1 or 2 HNPCC FAP PALB2	Smoking, exposure to benzenes or other carcinogens	1 or more FDR with PC	New adult-onset diabetes, unexplained weight loss, epigastric or interscapular pain, malabsorption

candidates, and cost-effective analysis currently suggests that screening individuals more than 70 years of age can be an expensive strategy.[4]

Who Should Be Doing Screening?

Consensus exists that screening should take place at high-volume, multidisciplinary centers, ideally within an active research study. The goal of these screening programs should be identification of high-risk lesions amenable to surgical resection. In general, high-risk lesions are identified as PanIN-3, IPMN with high-grade dysplasia, and stage I (T1N0M0) pancreatic cancer.[59] However, controversy remains concerning the optimal imaging modalities used for screening and how best to manage identified lesions.

How Should Patients Be Screened?

Serologic testing

Serologic testing for early detection of pancreatic cancer remains elusive. Several biomarkers have been evaluated, most notably CA19-9. However, no test has had adequate sensitivity or specificity for screening average-risk populations. CA19-9 has been used as an initial screening test in one feasibility study of 546 individuals with at least 1 family member with pancreatic cancer. If CA 19-9 returned greater than 37 U/mL, patients subsequently underwent evaluation with endoscopic ultrasound. In this study, 1 pancreatic adenocarcinoma (T2N0M0) and 4 other pancreatic lesions (neuroendocrine tumor, PanIN-1, MCN, IPMN) were identified, resulting in a reported diagnostic yield of 0.9% (5/546) for pancreatic neoplasia and 0.2% yield for pancreatic adenocarcinoma.[60] The diagnostic yield for pancreatic neoplasia of this screening test is lower than that of other reported screening trials; however, the diagnostic yield of detecting an asymptomatic high-risk lesion is on par with several trials (**Table 4**). Other studies have not found CA19-9 to be useful in the early detection of pancreatic neoplasia in FPC kindreds.[50,61,62]

Testing high-risk patients for glucose intolerance may help identify patients at risk for pancreatic cancer.[63] In our experience, 50% of patients with an abnormal EUS had glucose intolerance, whereas only 17% of patients with normal EUS had glucose intolerance, and 60% of individuals with histologically proven PanIN or cancer have glucose intolerance (Brentnall, unpublished data). To our knowledge, this finding has yet to be examined outside our institution and awaits further study.

Imaging

Currently EUS and/or MRI are the most commonly used modalities for pancreatic cancer screening. Computed tomography (CT) and MRI find incidental cysts in 2.4% and 2.8% of the general population, respectively.[64,65] In high-risk individuals, the incidence of pancreatic lesions has been reported from 8.3% to 76%.[49,66]

To date, 4 studies have reported the use of MRI plus or minus MRCP[49,51,58,61] and 5 studies have reported EUS as an initial screening test.[44,50,57,62,66,67] Canto and colleagues[66] recently published their prospective work comparing imaging modalities in 216 high-risk individuals. MRI/MRCP and EUS outperformed CT in the ability to detect any cystic or solid lesions, identifying 77% (MRI/MRCP) and 79% (EUS) of detected lesions compared with only 13.8% (CT). The concordance between EUS and MRI/MRCP was 91%. MRI and EUS detected subcentimeter cysts in 33% and 36% of patients with FPC, respectively.[66] Given the need for frequent surveillance and the risk of radiation, CT is not used in current screening protocols.

High-risk patients also have chronic pancreatitis type changes on EUS. Between 14% and 60% of high-risk patients have been described to have parenchymal changes, including hyperechoic stranding, hypoechoic lobules, and echogenic duct-walls.[44,50,66] On resection, these pancreata typically show lobular atrophy, exuberant fibroblast growth, and cystic changes in the tertiary ducts in the setting of PanIN and IPMN; these histologic changes of fibrosis and cystic lesions likely underlie the EUS image findings.[36,68,69] Some posit that PanIN and IPMN may cause local ductal obstruction and inflammation, which further precipitate lobular atrophy and the chronic inflammatory change seen on EUS.[36] Although EUS remains the most accurate imaging to detect parenchymal and small duct dilatation of the pancreas, it is also a highly subjective test. Despite a consensus working group, endoscopic impression of these changes is operator dependent.[70]

Usually when one imaging test is abnormal in high-risk individuals, a second confirmatory imaging test is performed. Two of the larger US cohort studies to date (the cancer of the pancreas consortium [CAPS] protocol led by M. Canto and the Seattle studies led by T. Brentnall) use EUS as the initial imaging test, followed by pancreatogram for validation. To better evaluate the ductal extent of worrisome EUS findings, the Seattle protocol often uses endoscopic retrograde pancreatogram (ERP) to better detail the abnormalities in the secondary pancreatic ducts such as saccular dilations, which are associated with high-grade PanIN lesions.[50] In this protocol, ERP has resulted in less than 3% risk of pancreatitis from the procedure. In contrast, the CAPS protocol uses MRCP because of concerns for ERP-related pancreatitis. The two programs have differences in the type of incipient lesions discovered at pancreatic resection: IPMN lesions are more common in the CAPS program, whereas PanIN-3 is more common in resected pancreata from the Seattle protocol. Whether this represents a difference in the imaging approaches that eventually lead to surgery or whether there are differences in the two cohorts remains to be seen.

Because of increased extrapancreatic cancer-related mortality,[8,17,18] cross-sectional imaging may find additional primary malignancies. However, in reported screening on 1054 high-risk individuals (HRI), only 17 nonpancreatic neoplasms were found (1.6% yield), of which 6 were benign neoplasms. This low yield may be caused by the limited nature of abdominal MRI in diagnosing breast, skin, lung, or colorectal cancer.

Table 4
Diagnostic yield of reported pancreatic cancer screening programs

Study	N	Screening Modality	Follow-up Reported	Diagnostic Yield (%)	Surgical Resection (%)	Pancreatic Cancer	High-grade Neoplasm: Dysplasia or IPMN	Low-grade Neoplasm: Dysplasia or IPMN	Other Pancreatic Neoplasm	Successful Yield[a] (%)
Kimmy et al,[71] 2002	46	EUS ± ERP/MRCP	Mean 5 y	13/46 (28)	12/46 (26)	—	8 PanIN-3	4 PanIN-2	—	8/46 (17)
Canto et al,[57] 2004	38	EUS	Mean 22 mo	29/38 (76)	7/38 (18.4)	1 stage IIb	1 PanIN-1 to PanIN-3	1 IPMN, 6 PanIN-1 to PanIN-2	3 SCA	1/38 (2.6)
Canto et al,[44] 2006	78	EUS	12 mo	17/78 (22)	7/78 (10.2)	1 stage IV	2 PanIN-3, 1 HG IPMN	5 LG IPMN, 2 PanIN-1 to PanIN-2	—	3/78 (3.8)
Poley et al,[67] 2009	44	EUS	First-time screen	10/44 (23)	3/44 (6.8)	2 stage IIb, 1 stage I	—	—	—	1/44 (2.3)
Langer et al,[62] 2009	76	EUS + MRI + MRCP	Median 2 examinations	28/76 (36)	7/76 (9.2)	—	—	1 LG IPMN, 1 PanIN-1, 1 PanIN-2	3 SCA	0/76 (0)
Verna et al,[61] 2010	51	EUS ± MRI/MRCP	First-time screen	20/51 (39)	6/51 (11.8)	1 stage IV, 1 stage Ib	—	4 PanIN-2, 3 LG IPMN	—	0/51 (0)

Ludwig et al,[49] 2011	109	MRCP + EUS (+FNA)	12 mo	9/109 (8.3)	6/109 (6.4)	1 stage IIa	1 PanIN-3	3 PanIN-1 to PanIN-2, LG IPMN	—	1/109 (0.9)
Vasen et al,[58] 2011	79	MRI + MRCP	4 y	16/79 (20)	7/79 (10)	7 PC (2 stage Ia)	—	2 PanIN-2	—	2/79 (2.5)
Zubarik et al,[60] 2011	546	CA 19-9	First-time screen	5/546 (0.9)	3/546 (0.5)	1 stage IIb	—	1 PanIN-1	1 NET	0/546 (0)
Al Sukhni et al,[72] 2012	262	MRI	Mean 4.2 y	84/262 (32)	4/262 (1.5)	2 stage IV, 1 stage IIb	—	1 PanIN-1 to PanIN-2, 1 LG IPMN	—	0/262 (0)
Canto et al,[59,66] 2012	216	MRI, EUS, CT	12 mo	92/216 (42.6)	5/216 (2.3)	—	1 MD-IPMN with HGD and multiple PanIN-1–3, 1 MD-IPMN, 1 PanIN-3	2 PanIN-1 to PanIN-2	1 NET	3/216 (1.4)
Totals	—	—	—	323/1545 (21)	67/1545 (4)	19	—	—	—	19/1545 (1.2)

Diagnostic yield: percentage of patients with a pancreatic lesion found using screening modality.

Abbreviations: HG, high grade; HGD, high grade dysplasia; IPMN, intraductal pancreatic mucinous neoplasm; LG, low grade; NET, neuroendocrine tumor; PC, pancreatic cancer; SCA, serous cystadenoma.

[a] Successful yield is surgical resection of PanIN-3, high-grade IPMN, or T1N0M0 disease.

Frequency of Imaging

Each consecutive imaging study is typically compared with the baseline when looking for changes in the pancreas over time. Many programs recommend annual imaging for high-risk individuals from FPC kindreds. This interval may be shortened or lengthened according to the extent of abnormalities noted at the study, the symptoms of the patient, and/or other moderating factors.

How Should Suspect Lesions Be Managed?

The published screening studies clearly show that evaluation of high-risk individuals with EUS and MRI results in new diagnoses of neoplastic lesions. Two issues are central to the management of such neoplastic lesions in the setting of FPC: (1) IPMN and PanIN lesions can be multifocal-interspersed throughout the pancreatic gland; and (2) waiting for masses or confirmed cancer to form is often associated with metastatic disease. For this reason, many investigators currently target PanIN-3 or IPMN with high-grade dysplasia as diagnostic criteria that would merit surgery. The CAPS group has proposed surgical management of solitary masses, suspected main duct or mixed IPMN, branch-duct IPMN greater than 2 cm and/or with concerning features such as mural nodules, and abnormal cytology.[66] Management of high-risk individuals who have high-grade PanIN is more challenging, because the imaging changes in PanIN-3 can be subtler than the cystic lesions associate with IPMN. Thus, in the absence of masses or cystic lesions, the diagnosis of PanIN-3 must be made through a tissue diagnosis. Given the multifocal nature of the PanIN-3 disease in FPC, total pancreatectomy is definitive therapy; however, this results in brittle diabetes. In the Seattle protocol, high-risk individuals with changes consistent with chronic pancreatitis on EUS, abnormal ductal changes on ERP/MRP, and multifocal PanIN-3 documented on pancreatic resection are offered total pancreatectomy if the individual is in robust health. Those who have PanIN-1 to PanIN-2 or other benign disease continue annual surveillance. Other institutions have advocated for partial pancreatectomy of all high-risk lesions, with continued surveillance for progression.[51,57,58,61,66,67] An additional concern, which may be addressed with future study, is how postsurgical change complicates further surveillance of the remnant organ in high-risk individuals.

Accepting the large amount of heterogeneity in studies, of the 1513 individuals screened by EUS and/or MRI, 21% (n = 317) had a clinically relevant lesion as defined by their research protocol (see **Table 4**). Of these individuals, 62 surgeries were performed and pancreatic cancer was found in 30% of the operated patients (n = 19/62). Most discovered cancers were stage II or more advanced; 5 had metastatic disease and only 3 had T1N0M0 disease. When specifically concerned with detecting and removing high-risk lesions (early stage PC, PanIN-3, IPMN with high-grade dysplasia), 29% of the operated patients (n = 18/62) had successful resection. The programs that had the most success in detecting early stage cancer, PanIN-3, and IPMN with high-grade dysplasia were those that use a combination of EUS and MRI/MRCP/or ERP. Programs that relied only on MRI or MRCP had more individuals diagnosed with later-stage cancers. These findings suggest that a combination of imaging studies that include EUS may be more sensitive in detecting curable disease; however, further analysis using uniform imaging protocols would need to be performed to validate this conjecture.

The natural history of neoplastic progression and timing of surgery are topics that need further evidenced-based research, but the studies to date provide valuable information suggesting that waiting for masses/cancer to form can lead to metastatic and incurable disease. Only 3 of 19 discovered cancers were T1N0M0, which underscores the need to identify incipient disease at its highest grade of precancer. Strategies that help identify PanIN-3 and IPMN with high-grade dysplasia are warranted; surgical or medical management at this earlier stage of disease may help prevent later-stage, incurable adenocarcinoma. In addition, further risk stratification of patients with FPC to identify those who require the closest surveillance would be useful to appropriate health care resources in the most cost-effective manner.

SUMMARY

Despite a lack of a universally accepted screening protocol, surveillance using EUS plus/minus MRI/MRCP is well tolerated and, for individuals at high risk for pancreatic cancer, screening can find precancerous and early stage disease. Thus far, the use of CA 19–9, CT, or MRI as a single imaging modality has proved low yield in the detection of early curable disease. However, it is hoped that longer-term data will clarify the best imaging modality, or combination of imaging modalities, and the timing of first-time screening and age to stop screening. Further research is also needed to clarify the natural history of PanIN (time to progression, risk factors, and imaging characteristics) to ensure the successful management of high-risk individuals.

REFERENCES

1. Siegel R, Naishadham D, Jemal A. Cancer statistics, 2012. CA Cancer J Clin 2012;62(1):10–29. http://dx.doi.org/10.3322/caac.20138.
2. Shimizu Y, Yasui K, Matsueda K, et al. Small carcinoma of the pancreas is curable: new computed tomography finding, pathological study and postoperative results from a single institute. J Gastroenterol Hepatol 2005;20(10):1591–4. http://dx.doi.org/10.1111/j.1440-1746.2005.03895.x.
3. Yeo CJ, Cameron JL. Prognostic factors in ductal pancreatic cancer. Langenbecks Arch Surg 1998;383(2):129–33.
4. Rulyak SJ, Kimmey MB, Veenstra DL, et al. Cost-effectiveness of pancreatic cancer screening in familial pancreatic cancer kindreds. Gastrointest Endosc 2003; 57(1):23–9. http://dx.doi.org/10.1067/mge.2003.28.
5. Hruban RH, Canto MI, Goggins M, et al. Update on familial pancreatic cancer. Adv Surg 2010;44:293–311.
6. Bartsch DK, Gress TM, Langer P. Familial pancreatic cancer-current knowledge. Nat Rev Gastroenterol Hepatol 2012;9(8):445–53. http://dx.doi.org/10.1038/nrgastro.2012.111.
7. Klein AP, Brune KA, Petersen GM, et al. Prospective risk of pancreatic cancer in familial pancreatic cancer kindreds. Cancer Res 2004;64(7):2634–8.
8. Schneider R, Slater EP, Sina M, et al. German national case collection for familial pancreatic cancer (FaPaCa): ten years experience. Fam Cancer 2011;10(2): 323–30. http://dx.doi.org/10.1007/s10689-010-9414-x.
9. Tersmette AC, Petersen GM, Offerhaus GJ, et al. Increased risk of incident pancreatic cancer among first-degree relatives of patients with familial pancreatic cancer. Clin Cancer Res 2001;7(3):738–44.
10. Applebaum SE, Kant JA, Whitcomb DC, et al. Genetic testing. Counseling, laboratory, and regulatory issues and the EUROPAC protocol for ethical research in multicenter studies of inherited pancreatic diseases. Med Clin North Am 2000; 84(3):575–88, viii.
11. Audibert A, Rufat P, Maire F, et al. Incidence of pancreatic and extra-pancreatic cancers in the families of patients with pancreatic adenocarcinoma: results of prospective survey. Pancreatology 2002;2:256.

12. Klein AP, Beaty TH, Bailey-Wilson JE, et al. Evidence for a major gene influencing risk of pancreatic cancer. Genet Epidemiol 2002;23(2):133–49. http://dx.doi.org/10.1002/gepi.1102.
13. Petersen GM, Amundadottir L, Fuchs CS, et al. A genome-wide association study identifies pancreatic cancer susceptibility loci on chromosomes 13q22.1, 1q32.1 and 5p15.33. Nat Genet 2010;42(3):224–8. http://dx.doi.org/10.1038/ng.522.
14. Brentnall TA, Lai LA, Coleman J, et al. Arousal of cancer-associated stroma: over-expression of palladin activates fibroblasts to promote tumor invasion. PLoS One 2012;7(1):e30219. http://dx.doi.org/10.1371/journal.pone.0030219.
15. McFaul CD, Greenhalf W, Earl J, et al. Anticipation in familial pancreatic cancer. Gut 2006;55(2):252–8. http://dx.doi.org/10.1136/gut.2005.065045.
16. Brune KA, Lau B, Palmisano E, et al. Importance of age of onset in pancreatic cancer kindreds. J Natl Cancer Inst 2010;102(2):119–26. http://dx.doi.org/10.1093/jnci/djp466.
17. Hemminki K, Li X. Familial and second primary pancreatic cancers: a nationwide epidemiologic study from Sweden. Int J Cancer 2003;103(4):525–30. http://dx.doi.org/10.1002/ijc.10863.
18. Wang L, Brune KA, Visvanathan K, et al. Elevated cancer mortality in the relatives of patients with pancreatic cancer. Cancer Epidemiol Biomarkers Prev 2009;18(11):2829–34. http://dx.doi.org/10.1158/1055-9965.EPI-09-0557.
19. Giardiello FM, Offerhaus GJ, Lee DH, et al. Increased risk of thyroid and pancreatic carcinoma in familial adenomatous polyposis. Gut 1993;34(10):1394–6.
20. Giardiello FM, Welsh SB, Hamilton SR, et al. Increased risk of cancer in the Peutz-Jeghers syndrome. N Engl J Med 1987;316(24):1511–4. http://dx.doi.org/10.1056/NEJM198706113162404.
21. Brand RE, Lerch MM, Rubinstein WS, et al. Advances in counselling and surveillance of patients at risk for pancreatic cancer. Gut 2007;56(10):1460–9. http://dx.doi.org/10.1136/gut.2006.108456.
22. Rulyak SJ, Lowenfels AB, Maisonneuve P, et al. Risk factors for the development of pancreatic cancer in familial pancreatic cancer kindreds. Gastroenterology 2003;124(5):1292–9.
23. Prokopczyk B, Hoffmann D, Bologna M, et al. Identification of tobacco-derived compounds in human pancreatic juice. Chem Res Toxicol 2002;15(5):677–85.
24. Huxley R, Ansary-Moghaddam A, Berrington de Gonzalez A, et al. Type-II diabetes and pancreatic cancer: a meta-analysis of 36 studies. Br J Cancer 2005;92(11):2076–83. http://dx.doi.org/10.1038/sj.bjc.6602619.
25. Lynch SM, Vrieling A, Lubin JH, et al. Cigarette smoking and pancreatic cancer: a pooled analysis from the pancreatic cancer cohort consortium. Am J Epidemiol 2009;170(4):403–13. http://dx.doi.org/10.1093/aje/kwp134.
26. Wang W, Chen S, Brune KA, et al. PancPRO: risk assessment for individuals with a family history of pancreatic cancer. J Clin Oncol 2007;25(11):1417–22. http://dx.doi.org/10.1200/JCO.2006.09.2452.
27. Hruban RH, Maitra A, Goggins M. Update on pancreatic intraepithelial neoplasia. Int J Clin Exp Pathol 2008;1(4):306–16.
28. Hruban RH, Takaori K, Klimstra DS, et al. An illustrated consensus on the classification of pancreatic intraepithelial neoplasia and intraductal papillary mucinous neoplasms. Am J Surg Pathol 2004;28(8):977–87.
29. Macgregor-Das AM, Iacobuzio-Donahue CA. Molecular pathways in pancreatic carcinogenesis. J Surg Oncol 2012. http://dx.doi.org/10.1002/jso.23213.
30. Baumgart M, Heinmoller E, Horstmann O, et al. The genetic basis of sporadic pancreatic cancer. Cell Oncol 2005;27(1):3–13.

31. Brune K, Hong SM, Li A, et al. Genetic and epigenetic alterations of familial pancreatic cancers. Cancer Epidemiol Biomarkers Prev 2008;17(12):3536–42. http://dx.doi.org/10.1158/1055-9965.EPI-08-0630.

32. Crnogorac-Jurcevic T, Chelala C, Barry S, et al. Molecular analysis of precursor lesions in familial pancreatic cancer. PLoS One 2013;8(1):e54830.

33. Andea A, Sarkar F, Adsay VN. Clinicopathological correlates of pancreatic intra-epithelial neoplasia: a comparative analysis of 82 cases with and 152 cases without pancreatic ductal adenocarcinoma. Mod Pathol 2003;16(10):996–1006. http://dx.doi.org/10.1097/01.MP.0000087422.24733.62.

34. Schwartz AM, Henson DE. Familial and sporadic pancreatic carcinoma, epidemiologic concordance. Am J Surg Pathol 2007;31(4):645–6. http://dx.doi.org/10.1097/PAS.0b013e31802d6d42.

35. Shi C, Klein AP, Goggins M, et al. Increased prevalence of precursor lesions in familial pancreatic cancer patients. Clin Cancer Res 2009;15(24):7737–43. http://dx.doi.org/10.1158/1078-0432.CCR-09-0004.

36. Brune K, Abe T, Canto M, et al. Multifocal neoplastic precursor lesions associated with lobular atrophy of the pancreas in patients having a strong family history of pancreatic cancer. Am J Surg Pathol 2006;30(9):1067–76.

37. Terhune PG, Phifer DM, Tosteson TD, et al. K-ras mutation in focal proliferative lesions of human pancreas. Cancer Epidemiol Biomarkers Prev 1998;7(6):515–21.

38. Lindgren G, Liljegren A, Jaramillo E, et al. Adenoma prevalence and cancer risk in familial non-polyposis colorectal cancer. Gut 2002;50(2):228–34.

39. Sohn TA, Yeo CJ, Cameron JL, et al. Intraductal papillary mucinous neoplasms of the pancreas: an updated experience. Ann Surg 2004;239(6):788–97 [discussion: 797–9].

40. Abe T, Fukushima N, Brune K, et al. Genome-wide allelotypes of familial pancreatic adenocarcinomas and familial and sporadic intraductal papillary mucinous neoplasms. Clin Cancer Res 2007;13(20):6019–25. http://dx.doi.org/10.1158/1078-0432.CCR-07-0471.

41. Luttges J, Zamboni G, Longnecker D, et al. The immunohistochemical mucin expression pattern distinguishes different types of intraductal papillary mucinous neoplasms of the pancreas and determines their relationship to mucinous non-cystic carcinoma and ductal adenocarcinoma. Am J Surg Pathol 2001;25(7):942–8.

42. Maguchi H, Tanno S, Mizuno N, et al. Natural history of branch duct intraductal papillary mucinous neoplasms of the pancreas: a multicenter study in Japan. Pancreas 2011;40(3):364–70. http://dx.doi.org/10.1097/MPA.0b013e31820a5975.

43. Rebours V, Couvelard A, Peyroux JL, et al. Familial intraductal papillary mucinous neoplasms of the pancreas. Dig Liver Dis 2012;44(5):442–6. http://dx.doi.org/10.1016/j.dld.2011.07.003.

44. Canto MI, Goggins M, Hruban RH, et al. Screening for early pancreatic neoplasia in high-risk individuals: a prospective controlled study. Clin Gastroenterol Hepatol 2006;4(6):766–81. http://dx.doi.org/10.1016/j.cgh.2006.02.005 [quiz: 665].

45. Nehra D, Oyarvide VM, Mino-Kenudson M, et al. Intraductal papillary mucinous neoplasms: does a family history of pancreatic cancer matter? Pancreatology 2012;12(4):358–63. http://dx.doi.org/10.1016/j.pan.2012.05.011.

46. Lubezky N, Ben-Haim M, Lahat G, et al. Intraductal papillary mucinous neoplasm of the pancreas: associated cancers, family history, genetic predisposition? Surgery 2012;151(1):70–5. http://dx.doi.org/10.1016/j.surg.2011.06.036.

47. Cubilla AL, Fitzgerald PJ. Morphological lesions associated with human primary invasive nonendocrine pancreas cancer. Cancer Res 1976;36(7 Pt 2):2690–8.

48. Pour PM, Sayed S, Sayed G. Hyperplastic, preneoplastic and neoplastic lesions found in 83 human pancreases. Am J Clin Pathol 1982;77(2):137–52.
49. Ludwig E, Olson SH, Bayuga S, et al. Feasibility and yield of screening in relatives from familial pancreatic cancer families. Am J Gastroenterol 2011;106(5):946–54. http://dx.doi.org/10.1038/ajg.2011.65.
50. Brentnall TA, Bronner MP, Byrd DR, et al. Early diagnosis and treatment of pancreatic dysplasia in patients with a family history of pancreatic cancer. Ann Intern Med 1999;131(4):247–55.
51. Al-Sukhni W, Borgida A, Rothenmund H, et al. Screening for pancreatic cancer in a high-risk cohort: an eight-year experience. J Gastrointest Surg 2012;16(4): 771–83. http://dx.doi.org/10.1007/s11605-011-1781-6.
52. Brat DJ, Lillemoe KD, Yeo CJ, et al. Progression of pancreatic intraductal neoplasias to infiltrating adenocarcinoma of the pancreas. Am J Surg Pathol 1998;22(2): 163–9.
53. Harinck F, Nagtegaal T, Kluijt I, et al. Feasibility of a pancreatic cancer surveillance program from a psychological point of view. Genet Med 2011;13(12): 1015–24. http://dx.doi.org/10.1097/GIM.0b013e31822934f5.
54. Hart SL, Torbit LA, Crangle CJ, et al. Moderators of cancer-related distress and worry after a pancreatic cancer genetic counseling and screening intervention. Psychooncology 2011. http://dx.doi.org/10.1002/pon.2026.
55. Maheu C, Vodermaier A, Rothenmund H, et al. Pancreatic cancer risk counselling and screening: impact on perceived risk and psychological functioning. Fam Cancer 2010;9(4):617–24. http://dx.doi.org/10.1007/s10689-010-9354-5.
56. Kimmey MB, Bronner MP, Byrd DR, et al. Screening and surveillance for hereditary pancreatic cancer. Gastrointest Endosc 2002;56(Suppl 4):S82–6.
57. Canto MI, Goggins M, Yeo CJ, et al. Screening for pancreatic neoplasia in high-risk individuals: an EUS-based approach. Clin Gastroenterol Hepatol 2004;2(7): 606–21.
58. Vasen HF, Wasser M, van Mil A, et al. Magnetic resonance imaging surveillance detects early-stage pancreatic cancer in carriers of a p16-leiden mutation. Gastroenterology 2011;140(3):850–6. http://dx.doi.org/10.1053/j.gastro.2010.11.048.
59. Canto MI, Harinck F, Hruban RH, et al. International Cancer of the Pancreas Screening (CAPS) Consortium summit on the management of patients with increased risk for familial pancreatic cancer. Gut 2012. http://dx.doi.org/10.1136/gutjnl-2012-303108.
60. Zubarik R, Gordon SR, Lidofsky SD, et al. Screening for pancreatic cancer in a high-risk population with serum CA 19-9 and targeted EUS: a feasibility study. Gastrointest Endosc 2011;74(1):87–95. http://dx.doi.org/10.1016/j.gie.2011.03.1235.
61. Verna EC, Hwang C, Stevens PD, et al. Pancreatic cancer screening in a prospective cohort of high-risk patients: a comprehensive strategy of imaging and genetics. Clin Cancer Res 2010;16(20):5028–37. http://dx.doi.org/10.1158/1078-0432.CCR-09-3209.
62. Langer P, Kann PH, Fendrich V, et al. Five years of prospective screening of high-risk individuals from families with familial pancreatic cancer. Gut 2009;58(10): 1410–8. http://dx.doi.org/10.1136/gut.2008.171611.
63. Pannala R, Leibson CL, Rabe KG, et al. Temporal association of changes in fasting blood glucose and body mass index with diagnosis of pancreatic cancer. Am J Gastroenterol 2009;104(9):2318–25. http://dx.doi.org/10.1038/ajg.2009.253.
64. Laffan TA, Horton KM, Klein AP, et al. Prevalence of unsuspected pancreatic cysts on MDCT. AJR Am J Roentgenol 2008;191(3):802–7. http://dx.doi.org/10.2214/AJR.07.3340.

65. de Jong K, Nio CY, Hermans JJ, et al. High prevalence of pancreatic cysts detected by screening magnetic resonance imaging examinations. Clin Gastroenterol Hepatol 2010;8(9):806–11. http://dx.doi.org/10.1016/j.cgh.2010.05.017.

66. Canto MI, Hruban RH, Fishman EK, et al. Frequent detection of pancreatic lesions in asymptomatic high-risk individuals. Gastroenterology 2012;142(4):796–804. http://dx.doi.org/10.1053/j.gastro.2012.01.005 [quiz: e14–5].

67. Poley JW, Kluijt I, Gouma DJ, et al. The yield of first-time endoscopic ultrasonography in screening individuals at a high risk of developing pancreatic cancer. Am J Gastroenterol 2009;104(9):2175–81. http://dx.doi.org/10.1038/ajg.2009.276.

68. Aimoto T, Uchida E, Nakamura Y, et al. Multicentric pancreatic intraepithelial neoplasias (PanINs) presenting with the clinical features of chronic pancreatitis. J Hepatobiliary Pancreat Surg 2008;15(5):549–53. http://dx.doi.org/10.1007/s00534-007-1269-7.

69. Takaori K, Matsusue S, Fujikawa T, et al. Carcinoma in situ of the pancreas associated with localized fibrosis: a clue to early detection of neoplastic lesions arising from pancreatic ducts. Pancreas 1998;17(1):102–5.

70. Topazian M, Enders F, Kimmey M, et al. Interobserver agreement for EUS findings in familial pancreatic-cancer kindreds. Gastrointest Endosc 2007;66(1):62–7. http://dx.doi.org/10.1016/j.gie.2006.09.018.

71. Kimmy MB, Bronner MP, Byrd DR, et al. Screening and surveillance for hereditary pancreatic cancer. Gastrointest Endosc 2002;56(4 Suppl):S82–6.

72. Al-Sukhni W, Borgida A, Rothenmund H, et al. J Gastrointest Surg 2012;16(4):771–83.

Resection Margins in Pancreatic Cancer

Caroline S. Verbeke, MD, PhD, FRCPath*

KEYWORDS

- Pancreatic cancer • Resection margin • Pancreatoduodenectomy • Pathology
- Survival

KEY POINTS

- The rate of microscopic margin involvement (R1 rate) for pancreatic cancer varies between published studies from less than 20% to more than 80%.
- The pathology examination procedure and in particular the specimen grossing technique have a significant impact on the accuracy of margin assessment.
- Recent studies report a consistently higher R1 rate (70% or more) if a novel grossing technique based on axial specimen dissection and extensive tissue sampling is used.
- The lack of consensus regarding terminology, definition of microscopic margin involvement, and pathology examination jeopardizes the validity of clinical trials that include surgical resection as a treatment arm for pancreatic cancer.
- The prognostic significance of microscopic margin involvement in pancreatic cancer is currently unknown.

INTRODUCTION

In recent years, there has been an increasing interest in the margin status of surgical resection specimens for ductal adenocarcinoma of the pancreas, both in terms of pathologic assessment and clinical implications. Although the reasons for this continued attention are multiple, it was mainly triggered by the introduction of a novel pathology examination technique for pancreatoduodenectomy specimens, which resulted in a significantly higher microscopic margin involvement rate (R1 rate) than when traditional grossing techniques were used.[1] In subsequent years the basic concepts of margin involvement in pancreatic cancer were critically reconsidered, as were the factors that influence the assessment of the margin status, and the implications of margin involvement regarding patient treatment and outcome. Although several

Funding Sources, Conflict of Interest: Nothing to disclose.
Division of Pathology, Department of Laboratory Medicine, Karolinska Institute, Karolinska University Hospital, Stockholm, Sweden
* Clinical Pathology and Cytology, F42, Karolinska University Hospital, Huddinge, Stockholm SE-141 86, Sweden.
E-mail address: caroline.verbeke@ki.se

questions remain unanswered and controversies continue to exist, it has become clear that the current disconcerting variety in reported R1 rates is to a large extent accounted for by divergence of pathology practice. This situation obviously raises concern regarding the appropriateness of the individual patient's management as well as the robustness of data from multicenter clinical trials.[2]

THE PROGNOSTIC SIGNIFICANCE OF MARGIN INVOLVEMENT

Ductal adenocarcinoma of the pancreas, commonly denoted as pancreatic cancer, has a poor prognosis, which is mainly a result of late clinical presentation and the limited effect of chemotherapy. In only 15% to 20% of patients is the tumor amenable to surgical resection, which increases the 5-year survival rate from less than 5% to 7%-25%.[3–5]

Numerous studies have identified multiple prognostic predictors, including tumor grade, lymph node metastasis, and perineural invasion.[6–10] The impact of microscopic margin involvement (R1) on overall and disease-free survival is not clear. The number of studies reporting a statistically significant prognostic impact of margin involvement[6,7,11–13] is comparable with that of reports on the lack of such a correlation.[4,14,15] However, the published R1 rates vary widely between studies, from less than 20% to more than 80% (**Table 1**), although patient-related and tumor-related characteristics are not significantly different, and all studies were undertaken in specialist pancreatic cancer centers, from which it can be presumed that surgery was performed according to current standards and preoperative patient selection followed comparable criteria.

The considerable divergence in R1 rate is not reflected in a comparably large difference in patient survival. The outcome of patients who underwent a complete resection

Table 1
Comparison of the rate of microscopic margin involvement (R1) and median survival after surgical resection of ductal adenocarcinoma of the pancreas between studies using the axial slicing technique or another grossing technique

Reference (Year)	Number of Patients	R1 Rate (%)	Median Survival R0	Median Survival R1
Axial Slicing Technique				
Verbeke et al,[1] 2006	54	85	37	11
Esposito et al,[16] 2008	111	76	—	—
Menon et al,[17] 2009	27	82	>55	14
Campbell et al,[18] 2009	163	79	25	15
Jamieson et al,[19] 2010	1848	74	26	15
Other Technique				
Willet et al,[20] 1993	72	51	20	12
Millikan et al,[21] 1999	84	29	17	8
Benassai et al,[22] 2000	75	20	17	9
Sohn et al,[6] 2000	616	30	12	19
Neoptolemos et al,[12] 2001	111	19	17	11
Raut et al,[15] 2007	360	17	28	22
Westgaard et al,[23] 2008	40	45	16	11
Hsu et al,[24] 2010	509	44	19	11
Gnerlich et al,[25] 2012	285	34	22	16

(R0) seems to be better in series with a high R1 rate than in studies with lower rates (see **Table 1**). These observations are difficult to explain by possible differences in patient selection or treatment. However, on close scrutiny of the methods section of the studies, it seems that those reporting a high R1 rate (>70%) were based on a novel pathology examination method,[1,16–19] whereas traditional methods had been used in studies with a lower R1 rate (17%–51%).[6,12,15,20–25] In addition, the studies differ in the number and location of the margins that had been included in the investigations, as well as in the diagnostic criteria that had been applied for the reporting of microscopic margin involvement. These differences highlight the controversies that exist regarding almost every aspect of margin assessment in pancreatic surgical resection specimens and in particular in those after pancreatoduodenectomy. The nature, causes, and consequences of these controversies are outlined in the following sections.

TERMINOLOGY

A recent study critically reviewing free-text histopathology reports found that 28 different names were used to describe various margins of pancreatoduodenectomy specimens.[26] This dissensus pertains only to the circumferential resection margins, whereas the terminology for the transection margins (of the stomach/proximal duodenum, distal duodenum, pancreatic neck and common bile duct) is universally accepted.

Fig. 1 shows the circumferential surfaces as these are distinguished in several countries and embedded in the national pathology guidelines of Sweden and the United Kingdom, for example.[27,28] The terminology is simple and based on anatomic localization or proximity to the superior mesenteric vessels. In particular, the surfaces facing the superior mesenteric artery (SMA) or vein (SMV) have been referred to by a variety

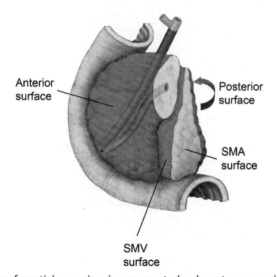

Anterior surface

Posterior surface

SMA surface

SMV surface

Fig. 1. The circumferential margins in pancreatoduodenectomy specimens consist of the anterior and posterior surfaces, as well as the surfaces facing the SMV and SMA. Color-coded inking of the surfaces allows identification of the individual margins during microscopic examination. Inked in purple is the circumferential soft tissue margin of the extrapancreatic common bile duct.

of terms, including retroperitoneal, uncinate, mesenteric, medial, and posterior. In some centers, the 'SMA margin' includes both the SMA-facing and SMV-facing surfaces, whereas in others the same term refers to the artery-facing margin only.

The circumferential resection margin of the soft tissue sheath around the extrapancreatic common bile duct stump (sometimes referred to as the radial periductal margin) is usually not considered in studies on pancreatic cancer. However, it is of importance for distal bile duct cancer involving the extrapancreatic segment of the bile duct.[29]

The lack of international consensus on the terminology for the circumferential resection margins is closely linked to a divergence in opinion and practice regarding the pathology assessment of these surfaces in terms of specimen dissection and tissue sampling.

GROSSING TECHNIQUES

Worldwide, a variety of grossing techniques for pancreatoduodenectomy specimens are used. The 3 main approaches differ in the plane of dissection and whether or not the pancreatic and bile duct are opened longitudinally. Specimen dissection is preceded by color-coded inking of the various surfaces of the pancreatoduodenectomy specimen, as shown in **Fig. 1**.

Bivalving and Multivalving Technique

For many decades, it has been traditional in pathology to open gastrointestinal cancer specimens longitudinally. Although this technique has now been abandoned in favor of cross sectioning of specimens from the tubular digestive tract, in some centers it continues being applied to pancreatoduodenectomy specimens. According to this technique, the main pancreatic duct and common bile duct are probed, and the specimen is sliced once or several times along the plane defined by both probes (**Fig. 2**). In this way, both ducts are exposed longitudinally in only 2 specimen slices facing the same dissection plane. This technique is challenging, not only when it comes to the insertion of probes into the narrow, distorted, or tumor-obstructed ducts but also regarding the subsequent slicing of the specimen along the probes. The resulting slices are large and require further dissection, which is usually performed by slicing in an additional, perpendicular plane,[30] as shown in **Fig. 2**. The use of different dissection planes, one of which varies between specimens depending on the configuration of the pancreatic and bile duct, hinders the pathologist's mental three-dimensional reconstruction of the tumor and its exact localization within the pancreatic head.

Bread Loaf Slicing Technique

According to this technique, the main pancreatic duct and common bile duct can be left untouched. Instead, the pancreatic head is serially sliced along a plane perpendicular to the longitudinal axis of the pancreatic neck (**Fig. 3**).[31] The main disadvantage of this technique is of a practical nature. The rubbery tubelike nature of the duodenum renders it difficult to slice the latter and the flanking pancreas in a longitudinal fashion, with the result that specimen slices through the ampulla and the junction with the pancreatic and common bile duct may be suboptimal (ie, incomplete, fragmented, or thicker than desired).

Serial slicing perpendicular to an axis that follows the curvature of the pancreatic head is advocated by the Japan Society of Pancreas.[32] It solves the practical problem mentioned earlier, but has the disadvantage that the sectioning is not parallel but fanlike and the resulting specimen slices are wedge-shaped rather than square.

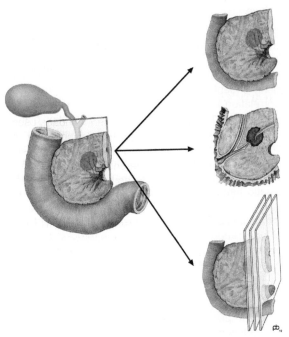

Fig. 2. Multivalve slicing along a plane defined by the main pancreatic duct and common bile duct results in several larger specimen slices, which usually require further dissection (as shown in *lower part*) to allow sampling of standard tissue blocks.

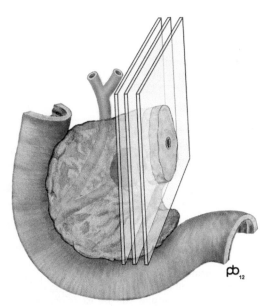

Fig. 3. With the bread loaf slicing technique, the pancreatic head is sliced in a plane perpendicular to the pancreatic neck.

Axial Slicing Technique

Following this technique, the specimen is sliced in an axial plane (ie, perpendicular to the longitudinal axis of the descending duodenum) (**Fig. 4**).[1] Slicing is easy to perform and results in many thin slices (on average 12 or more), which allow good views and from which it is easy to take tissue samples for microscopic examination. Because the axial dissection plane is identical to that of computed tomography or magnetic resonance imaging, correlation between pathology and imaging is straightforward and usually appreciated by the radiologists. Because the dissection plane is fixed (ie, independent of duct configuration, as is the case for the bivalving or multivalving technique), key anatomic structures such as the ampulla, common bile duct, and main pancreatic duct can be easily identified, since they always occur at the same position in the specimen slices. Regarding the assessment of the margin status, the entire surface of the pancreatic head can be inspected easily in every specimen slice (see **Fig. 4**).

The combination of these advantages allows not only exact identification of the three-dimensional localization and extension of the tumor in the specimen, it also facilitates detailed examination of the proximity of the tumor to the various resection margins, which is key to accurate margin assessment.

TISSUE SAMPLING

The extent of tissue sampling has a direct impact on the accuracy of the margin assessment.[1] If only a few samples are taken from the tumor and the nearest specimen surface, margin involvement risks being underestimated, because (unlike in

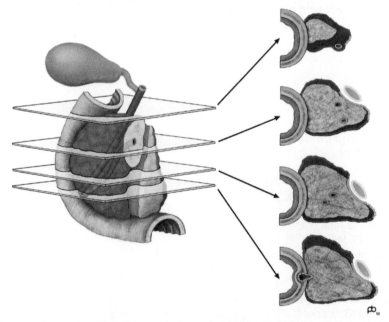

Fig. 4. According to the axial slicing technique, the pancreatic head is serially sectioned in a plane perpendicular to the longitudinal axis of the descending duodenum. In each of the specimen slices, the circumferential margins can be examined and the main pancreatic duct and common bile duct can be inspected over their entire course. The pale blue structure in the 3 lower specimen slices indicates the position of the SMV.

any other gastrointestinal cancer) the outline of pancreatic cancer is notoriously difficult to identify by macroscopic inspection. The reason for this situation is 2-fold. First, the periphery of the tumor is blurred by the chronic inflammation, pancreatic atrophy, and fibrosis that commonly accompany the cancer. Second, the growth of pancreatic cancer is characteristically highly dispersed, in particular at the invasive tumor front.[33] The tumor infiltrates surrounding nonneoplastic tissues in form of single cells or clusters rather than larger aggregates, and, not infrequently, tumor glands are devoid of associated stromal desmoplasia when invading the peripancreatic adipose tissue (so-called naked glands).[34] Because of both factors (the fibroinflammatory changes and the dispersed growth pattern), naked-eye identification of the invasive front of pancreatic cancer is commonly unreliable and inaccurate. Consequently, if tissue sampling is limited to areas of macroscopically unequivocal tumor growth, the highly infiltrative cancer cells at the tumor periphery are likely to remain undetected. This situation not only results in significant underestimation of tumor size and stage[35] but also bears the risk of underestimating margin involvement, because it is the tumor periphery, not the more readily visible tumor center, that jeopardizes the specimen margins.

In a discussion regarding tissue sampling for the assessment of resection margins, the limitations inherent to histopathology as a detection method should be kept in mind. Histopathology is poor when it comes to the identification of small structures (eg, a low number of pancreatic cancer cells) that are present (or of interest) only in a confined area (eg, the resection margin) that cannot be precisely targeted (eg, because of problematic macroscopic identification). Under these circumstances, the representativity of the tissue sections on which microscopic examination is based becomes the limiting factor. Standard tissue sections for microscopic examination, measuring approximately 2×1 cm in width and 5 μm in thickness, represent only a volume of 1 mm^3. If, for example, 2 standard tissue blocks are taken from a 1-cm-wide area that is macroscopically suspicious of margin involvement, only 1:1000 of the tissue of interest is examined. Consequently, even if microscopic examination of the 2 tissue sections reveals the presence of tumor cells at, for example, 1.5 mm from the specimen surface, and thus the margin status is by definition to be reported as R0, the exclusion value of margin involvement is low. Considering the dispersed growth pattern of pancreatic cancer, tumor cells may well be within 1 mm to the specimen margin (ie, fulfill the diagnostic criteria for R1), in the tissue levels above or below the sections that were submitted for microscopic examination.

The importance of extensive tissue sampling is further supported by a study that compared the detection rate of cancer cells in tissue from the peripancreatic circumferential resection margins based on K-ras mutational analysis versus conventional histology. In 43% of the cases that were negative on histology but positive according to K-ras analysis, cancer cells were identified when additional tissue sections were examined microscopically.[36]

The accuracy of margin assessment is to a significant degree determined during specimen grossing by the extent of tissue sampling and the dissection technique that is used, because the latter may be more or less conducive to meticulous macroscopic inspection.

DIAGNOSTIC CRITERIA OF MICROSCOPIC MARGIN INVOLVEMENT

Controversy exists regarding the diagnostic criteria for microscopic margin involvement. In many centers worldwide, tumor cells have to be present at the resection margin (0 mm clearance) for a diagnosis of R1 to be made. However, in other centers, particularly in Europe, a margin is regarded as involved if invasive tumor glands are

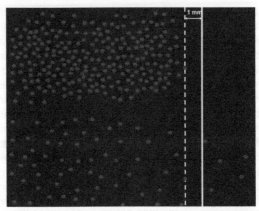

Fig. 5. The growth pattern of a cancer determines the minimum clearance on which the diagnosis of microscopic margin involvement (R1) is to be based. The red dots represent the tumor cells in cancers with a compact (*upper part*) and a more dispersed growth pattern (*lower part*). The yellow line indicates the surgical resection margin. The dotted white line indicates a clearance of 1 mm. Although for both tumors the minimum clearance is the same (ie, 1 mm), cells of the dispersedly growing cancer are left behind in the surgical bed (to the *right* of the *yellow line*), whereas resection of the compact-growing cancer is complete.

present within 1 mm to the resection margin. The latter definition is an adoption from rectal cancer, for which clinicopathologic studies reported an increased risk of local tumor recurrence if clearance to the margin is less than 1 mm.[37] Comparable data do not exist for pancreatic cancer. However, following simple theoretic considerations, an R1 definition based on 0 mm clearance seems unfounded in pancreatic cancer. As shown in **Fig. 5**, the 0-mm clearance definition is valid for tumors that grow in compact uninterrupted cell sheets. In contrast, in tumors growing in a less cohesive fashion such as rectal or pancreatic cancer, the absence of tumor cells

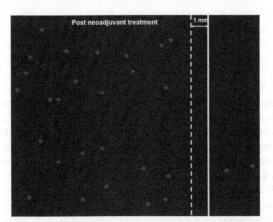

Fig. 6. Depiction of the same scenario as in **Fig. 5**, now after neoadjuvant treatment, which killed a proportion of the tumor cells. The growth pattern of both cancers is altered in a haphazard fashion. Overall, the distance between individual cells has increased. Although clearance to the resection margin is larger than before neoadjuvant treatment, a few widely scattered viable cells are left behind in the surgical bed (*lower part*).

immediately at the tissue surface (ie, 0 mm clearance) does not guarantee complete resection.

The more dispersed the tumor growth, the greater the clearance that is required to ensure that no cancer cells are left behind. Interesting in this respect is the recent morphometric evidence that the growth pattern of pancreatic cancer is considerably more dispersed than that of rectal cancer.[33] This finding implies that the R1 definition based on 1 mm clearance, as it is currently used for pancreatic cancer in some centers, is likely to overestimate complete resection. Pointing in the same direction, although investigated along entirely different lines, is the recent observation that the reporting of margin involvement based on 1.5 mm rather than 1 mm clearance results in improved prognostic stratification of patients who have pancreatic cancer.[38]

These considerations have particularly important implications for the assessment of microscopic margin involvement in pancreatic resection specimens after neoadjuvant treatment. The latter results in loss of viable tumor tissue, which depending on the success of the treatment, may vary considerably in extent.[39,40] In most patients, tumor regression is not complete, and the tumor persists in an apparently random distribution, whereby tumor cell singletons and clusters are scattered widely in highly atrophic and fibrotic pancreatic tissue. Thus, as a consequence of the treatment-induced tumor cell death, the original growth pattern of the tumor is lost, and the distance between residual tumor cells is overall considerably larger than in untreated tumor tissue (**Fig. 6**). This finding implies that reliable prediction of residual microscopic disease in the surgical bed is problematic, and that application of the conventional diagnostic criteria for R1 based on a minimum clearance of 1 mm leads to underestimation of residual disease. The results of a recent study confirm these theoretic considerations.[41] First, the analysis shows that after neoadjuvant chemoradiation, the clearance to the SMA-facing margin increases significantly ($\geq$10 mm in 39% of cases vs 19% of cases without neoadjuvant treatment). Second, the study also shows that after neoadjuvant treatment, the rate of local tumor recurrence does not differ between cases with clearance of 1 mm or less or more than 1 mm.

The assessment of the anterior pancreatic surface differs from that of the other circumferential resection margins. Because this is a free anatomic surface rather than a true surgical margin, the risk of residual tumor after surgical resection exists only if tumor cells breach this surface. Hence, the appropriate clearance to be observed for the anterior surface is 0 mm.

DIVERGENT INTERPRETATIONS OF R1

The significance of the mode of tumor spread at the specimen margins is a further point of controversy. Clearly, direct tumor growth up to or within 1 mm to the margin (depending on the R1 definition being used) is to be reported as R1. But does this also apply to tumor cells within blood vessels, lymphatics, perineural spaces, or lymph nodes?

There are no data on which to base a decision, but cases in which the margin is threatened only by the presence of tumor cells in any of the microscopic compartments mentioned earlier and not by direct invasion are rare.

One of the main problems underlying this controversy is the definition of R1. In daily clinical practice, R1 is commonly used synonymously with microscopic margin involvement, which is incorrect, because the R descriptor stands for residual disease, not resection margin.[42] According to the International Union Against Cancer (UICC), R1 is defined as 'microscopic residual disease'. This definition does not include stipulations regarding the site of the residual tumor cells or the mode of tumor propagation. Hence, for example, a microscopic tumor deposit detected in an aortocaval lymph node, or tumor cells en route along perineural clefts in the surgical bed, also represent microscopic residual disease (R1). From this observation, it follows that the meaning of R1 is closely linked with the risk of tumor recurrence, either local, regional, or distant.

However, in clinical practice, R1 has various meanings and connotations that differ from the original definition and lead to divergent implications in patient management. First and foremost, R1 is usually understood as a local phenomenon, in particular as an incomplete surgical resection, with tumor cells being left in the surgical bed and, consequently, with an increased risk of local recurrence. Whereas for many oncologists, the latter may prompt consideration of adjuvant treatment, others may feel discouraged to recommend chemotherapy in view of the alleged negative impact of margin involvement on the already poor outcome of patients who have pancreatic cancer.

Furthermore, the R status is commonly interpreted as an indicator of the quality of the surgery. However, recent studies have shown that the method and meticulousness of the pathology examination have a significant impact on margin status assessment,[1,16–19] and that 'in contrast to common belief, a high rate of R1 resections in pancreatic cancer is not a marker of low-quality surgery but rather of high-quality pathology.'[16] If surgery is performed according to standards of best practice, it seems that the R status is determined mainly by 3 factors: the extent and location of the tumor, and the meticulousness of the pathology examination.[43]

R0 and R1 are commonly used interchangeably with curative and noncurative. This lack of distinction between a microscopic finding and a denotation of expected treatment outcome adds to the confusion.

Uniform use and understanding of R0/R1 is urgently needed to allow unequivocal communication and clear reasoning, not the least about the implications of the R status in terms of patient treatment and outcome. The latter are outlined in more detail below.

R1 AND OVERALL OR DISEASE-FREE SURVIVAL

The impact of margin status on patient outcome remains controversial. Data regarding the correlation between microscopic margin involvement and survival are conflicting, which may not surprise given the presence of multiple confounding factors: differences in the pathology examination procedure, underpowered studies, and long study periods with a concomitant lack of diagnostic or therapeutic uniformity. A further important confounding factor is the misclassification of the cancer origin. Data in the literature indicate that distinction between pancreatic, ampullary, and distal bile duct cancer is not infrequently inaccurate and inconsistent (reviewed in Ref.[43]). Because the survival and R1 rate differ between these cancers, erroneous inclusion of ampullary and common bile duct cancers in pancreatic series is likely to result in obfuscation of key clinicopathologic data and identification of incorrect correlations with patient outcome.[44]

A further obstacle in the attempt at identifying the prognostic significance of margin involvement is the fact that most patients who suffer from pancreatic cancer have a full house of adverse prognostic factors (ie, advanced T stage, lymph node metastasis, and vascular and perineural invasion). Identification of the prognostic impact specifically related to margin involvement requires the analysis of prohibitively large case series.

While most studies concentrate on overall patient survival, comparatively few data are available regarding disease-free survival and its correlation with margin involvement. This situation may be because the site and time of tumor recurrence are often not well documented, because its development foreshadows limited survival and there is no agreed or effective treatment. Overall, 50% to more than 80% of patients with pancreatic cancer develop local tumor recurrence after a presumed R0 resection.[45–48] This observation implies that microscopic margin involvement is commonly underestimated, and suggests that the high R1 rates reported in recent studies may be more realistic. In all of these considerations, the impact of adjuvant treatment is difficult to judge, because it has not been administered uniformly, and results regarding its effectiveness are conflicting.[49–53]

However, in many, if not most, patients who have pancreatic cancer, it is the development of distant metastasis (usually in the liver) that determines survival, even in the presence of local tumor recurrence.[15,54] The full benefit of R0 resection may therefore be limited to patients without early distant relapse.

In view of the differences in pathology practice regarding the assessment of the margins in pancreatoduodenectomy specimens, it remains unknown whether the site of margin involvement has any bearing on outcome. In this respect, it is not surprising that preliminary results are conflicting: whereas in 1 study, the posterior margin was found to be the only site of R1 that influenced (disease-free) survival,[25] the transection margin of the pancreatic neck and the SMA-facing margin were the only prognostically significant sites of R1 according to another analysis.[19] There is no obvious reason why involvement of one margin should be of greater prognostic importance than that of another, except possibly that the density of lymphovascular channels and peripheral nerves differs between the various areas of peripancreatic soft tissue. The question of the prognostic significance of the site of margin involvement may be more of an academic interest, because if the pancreatoduodenectomy is performed according to current standards of best surgical practice, there is no scope for extended resection except (by a limited amount) of the pancreatic neck and common bile duct. Furthermore, because margin involvement is rarely the sole adverse factor, the site of margin involvement (even if found to be prognostically significant) is unlikely to influence postoperative treatment.

MACROSCOPIC MARGIN INVOLVEMENT (R2)

According to the UICC definition, R2 denotes the presence of macroscopic residual disease, without further indication of the site of the tumor residua.[42] In clinical practice, R2 usually refers to macroscopic residual tumor tissue at the resection margin, because the presence of gross tumor clearly outside the resection boundaries (eg, peritoneal or liver metastasis) represents a contraindication for surgery. The outcome of patients after an R2 resection is significantly worse than that of patients whose resection was reported as R1.[55] R2 resection usually suggests underestimation of local tumor extension and resectability on preoperative imaging. Discussion sometimes arises as to who should make an R2 diagnosis: the surgeon or the pathologist. Most commonly, the surgeon is aware that during resection gross tumor was left in situ, which is subsequently confirmed by the pathologist. Conversely, on rare occasions, after a presumed R0 resection, the pathologist may identify macroscopically visible tumor at the specimen margin and report the margin status as R2. However, this situation seems unfair, because the pathologist has better views than the surgeon on the margins after specimen fixation and dissection, and the advantage of microscopic confirmation. Therefore, in many pancreatic cancer centers, it is agreed that a diagnosis of R2 resection depends on the surgeon's assessment. In practice, it may be more objective and informative if the pathologist refrains from using the

R2 terminology, but instead states the extent over which the specimen surface is involved by tumor.

ISSUES TO BE ADDRESSED

The observation that divergence in terminology, definitions, and pathology practice leads to incomparability of R1 data is sobering. It highlights the need for urgent international consultation and agreement amongst surgeons, oncologists, and pathologists. Consensus regarding the terminology to denote the various surfaces of pancreatoduodenectomy specimens and the definition of microscopic margin involvement (ie, the minimum clearance) is a prerequisite for meaningful communication. Equally important is the international use of a standardized and rigorous pathology protocol for both the macroscopic and microscopic part of the examination. Although various guidelines for the reporting of pancreatic cancer specimens are available, they differ in aspects that affect the assessment of the margin status. Furthermore, some of these so-called guidelines are in fact minimum data sets, which list the data items that are to be included in the pathology report, but do not provide detailed guidance on how these key data should be obtained.[56]

Histopathology is the diagnostic gold standard for patients with pancreatic cancer who have undergone surgical resection. Hence, it is of paramount importance that quality assurance systems are in place to ensure the accuracy of the pathology data. Quality assurance is currently limited to slide review, and macroscopic examination is commonly excluded from this process, although during specimen grossing, important decisions are made regarding the location and origin of the cancer and its relationship to neighboring anatomic structures and the specimen margins. It is therefore essential that macroscopic findings can also be subjected to review for the purpose of second opinion or quality assurance. Close-up photographs of the specimen slices are a simple and effective way of ensuring that this decisive step in the diagnostic process can be reassessed.

These considerations regarding pathology quality assurance are essential for multicenter trials. Central review of both the macroscopic and microscopic findings along with a detailed pathology examination protocol should be integral parts of the trial procedure.

SUMMARY

The issue of margin involvement in pancreatic cancer surgery is controversially discussed. Both the R1 rate and the prognostic significance of microscopic margin involvement differ significantly between published series. However, in recent years, there has been a growing appreciation of the lack of consensus regarding conceptual as well as practical aspects of margin involvement and the assessment of the margin status. Central to the prevalent controversies is the lack of clarity about what R1 exactly stands for. The definition by the UICC (residual microscopic tumor) is possibly too general to be of practical and unequivocal use. It invites divergent interpretations and connotations and leads to varying practical implications in terms of patient management. The adherence to different criteria for the microscopic diagnosis of margin involvement, and the lack of uniformity in the terminology for the various margins of pancreatoduodenectomy specimens add to the confusion in this area. One of the most important causes for the conflicting results regarding margin status is the use of different pathology grossing procedures. Recent studies reported that the specimen dissection technique and extent of tissue sampling have an important impact on the accuracy of margin assessment. Axial specimen slicing, extensive tissue sampling, and multicolored inking of all specimen surfaces were shown to result in a significantly higher, more accurate R1 rate than when traditional grossing techniques are used. Only when international consensus on these various aspects of margin assessment is reached will pathology data on margin involvement be reliable and can multicenter clinical trials succeed in producing compelling data that allow optimal management of patients with pancreatic cancer.

ACKNOWLEDGMENTS

The author thanks Mr Paul Brown, Specialist Medical Illustrator, St James's University Hospital Leeds, for the color drawings.

REFERENCES

1. Verbeke CS, Leitch D, Menon KV, et al. Redefining the R1 resection in pancreatic cancer. Br J Surg 2006;93:1232–7.
2. Verbeke CS. Resection margins and R1 rates in pancreatic cancer: are we there yet? Histopathology 2008;52:787–96.
3. Jemal A, Siegel R, Ward E, et al. Cancer statistics, 2007. CA Cancer J Clin 2007; 57:43–66.
4. Schmidt CM, Powell ES, Yiannoutsos CT, et al. Pancreaticoduodenectomy: a 20-year experience in 516 patients. Arch Surg 2004;139:718–25.
5. Cameron JL, Riall TS, Coleman J, et al. One thousand consecutive pancreatico-duodenectomies. Ann Surg 2006;244:10–5.
6. Sohn TA, Yeo CJ, Cameron JL, et al. Resected adenocarcinoma of the pancreas–616 patients: results, outcomes, and prognostic indicators. J Gastrointest Surg 2000;4:567–79.
7. Winter JM, Cameron JL, Campbell KA, et al. 1423 pancreaticoduodenectomies for pancreatic cancer: a single-institution experience. J Gastrointest Surg 2006; 10:1199–210.
8. Wagner M, Redaelli C, Lietz M, et al. Curative resection is the single most important factor determining outcome in patients with pancreatic adenocarcinoma. Br J Surg 2004;91:586–94.
9. Lüttges J, Schemm S, Vogel I, et al. The grade of pancreatic ductal carcinoma is an independent prognostic factor and is superior to the immunohistochemical assessment of proliferation. J Pathol 2000;191:154–61.
10. Van Roest MH, Gouw AS, Peeters PM, et al. Results of pancreaticoduodenectomy in patients with periampullary adenocarcinoma: perineural growth more important prognostic factor than tumor localization. Ann Surg 2008;248: 97–103.
11. Yeo CJ, Cameron JL, Lillemoe KD, et al. Pancreaticoduodenectomy for cancer of the head of the pancreas: 201 patients. Ann Surg 1995;221:721–31.
12. Neoptolemos JP, Stocken DD, Dunn JA, et al. Influence of resection margins on survival for patients with pancreatic cancer treated by adjuvant chemoradiation and/or chemotherapy in the ESPAC-1 randomized controlled trial. Ann Surg 2001;234:758–68.
13. Jarufe NP, Coldham C, Mayer AD, et al. Favorable prognostic factors in a large UK experience of adenocarcinoma of the head of the pancreas and periampullary region. Dig Surg 2004;21:202–9.
14. Bouvet M, Gamagami RA, Gilpin EA, et al. Factors influencing survival after resection for periampullary neoplasms. Am J Surg 2000;180:13–7.

15. Raut CP, Tseng JF, Sun CC, et al. Impact of resection status on pattern of failure and survival after pancreaticoduodenectomy for pancreatic adenocarcinoma. Ann Surg 2007;246:52–60.
16. Esposito I, Kleeff J, Bergmann F, et al. Most pancreatic cancer resections are R1 resections. Ann Surg Oncol 2008;15:1651–60.
17. Menon KV, Gomez D, Smith AM, et al. Impact of margin status on survival following pancreatoduodenectomy for cancer: the Leeds Pathology Protocol (LEEPP). HPB (Oxford) 2009;11:18–24.
18. Campbell F, Smith RA, Whelan P, et al. Classification of R1 resections for pancreatic cancer: the prognostic relevance of tumour involvement within 1 mm of a resection margin. Histopathology 2009;55:277–83.
19. Jamieson NB, Foulis AK, Oien KA, et al. Positive immobilization margins alone do not influence survival following pancreatico-duodenectomy for pancreatic ductal adenocarcinoma. Ann Surg 2010;251:1003–10.
20. Willett CG, Lewandrowski K, Warschaw AL, et al. Resection margins in carcinoma of the head of the pancreas: implications for radiation therapy. Ann Surg 1993; 217:144–8.
21. Millikan KW, Deziel DJ, Silverstein JC, et al. Prognostic factors associated with resectable adenocarcinoma of the head of the pancreas. Am Surg 1999;65: 618–23.
22. Benassai G, Mastrorilli M, Quarto G, et al. Factors influencing survival after resection for ductal adenocarcinoma of the head of the pancreas. J Surg Oncol 2000; 73:212–8.
23. Westgaard A, Tafjord S, Farstad IN, et al. Resectable adenocarcinomas in the pancreatic head: the retroperitoneal resection margin is an independent prognostic factor. BMC Cancer 2008;8:5–15.
24. Hsu CC, Herman JM, Corsini MM, et al. Adjuvant chemoradiation for pancreatic adenocarcinoma: the Johns Hopkins Hospital-Mayo Clinic collaborative study. Ann Surg Oncol 2010;17:981–90.
25. Gnerlich JL, Luka SR, Deshpande AD, et al. Microscopic margins and patterns of treatment failure in resected pancreatic adenocarcinoma. Arch Surg 2012;147: 753–60.
26. Gill AJ, Johns AL, Eckstein R, et al. Synoptic reporting improves histopathological assessment of pancreatic resection specimens. Pathology 2009;41:161–7.
27. Björnstedt M, Franzén L, Glaumann H, et al. Gastrointestinal pathology–pancreas and peri-ampullary region. Recommendations from the KVAST Study Group of the Swedish Society for Pathology. Available at: http.//svfp.se/node/222. Accessed March 20, 2013.
28. The Royal College of Pathologists. Standards and datasets for reporting cancers. Dataset for the histopathological reporting of carcinomas of the pancreas, ampulla of Vater and common bile duct. 2nd edition. London: The Royal College of Pathologists; 2010.
29. Anthoney DA, Smith AM, Menon KM, et al. Distal bile duct cancer–clinicopathological features and prognostic factors. Pancreatology 2010;10:361.
30. Lüttges J, Zamboni G, Klöppel G. Recommendation for the examination of pancreaticoduodenectomy specimens removed from patients with carcinoma of the exocrine pancreas. A proposal for a standardized pathological staging of pancreaticoduodenectomy specimens including a checklist. Dig Dis 1999;16:291–6.
31. Hruban RH, Bishop Pitman M, Klimstra DS. Tumors of the pancreas. Atlas of tumor pathology, 4th Series, Fascicle 6. Washington, DC: Armed Forces Institute of Pathology; 2007.

32. Japan Pancreas Society. Classification of pancreatic cancer. 2nd edition. Tokyo: Kanehara; 2003.
33. Verbeke CS, Knapp J, Gladhaug IP. Tumour growth is more dispersed in pancreatic head cancers than in rectal cancer–implications for resection margin assessment. Histopathology 2011;59:1111–21.
34. Bandyopadhyay S, Basturk O, Coban I, et al. Isolated solitary ducts (naked ducts) in adipose tissue. A specific but underappreciated finding of pancreatic adenocarcinoma and one of the potential reasons of understaging and high recurrence rate. Am J Surg Pathol 2009;33:425–9.
35. Verbeke C, Sheridan M, Scarsbrook A, et al. How accurate is size assessment of pancreatic head cancers by radiology and pathology? Pancreatology 2010; 10:300.
36. Kim J, Reber HA, Dry SM, et al. Unfavourable prognosis associated with K-ras gene mutation in pancreatic cancer surgical margins. Gut 2006;55:1598–605.
37. Wibe A, Rendedal PR, Svensson E, et al. Prognostic significance of the circumferential resection margin following total mesorectal excision for rectal cancer. Br J Surg 2002;89:327–34.
38. Chang DK, Johns AL, Merrett ND, et al. Margin clearance and outcome in resected pancreatic cancer. J Clin Oncol 2009;27:2855–62.
39. Evans DE, Varadhachary GR, Crane CH, et al. Preoperative gemcitabine-based chemoradiation for patients with resectable adenocarcinoma of the pancreatic head. J Clin Oncol 2008;26:3496–502.
40. Chatterjee D, Katz MH, Rashid A, et al. Histologic grading the extent of residual carcinoma following neoadjuvant chemoradiation in pancreatic ductal adenocarcinoma. A predictor for patient outcome. Cancer 2011;118:3182–90.
41. Katz MH, Wang H, Balachandran A, et al. Effect of neoadjuvant chemoradiation and surgical technique on recurrence of localized pancreatic cancer. J Gastrointest Surg 2012;16:68–79.
42. Sobin LH, Gospodarowicz MK, Wittekind C, editors. UICC: TNM classification of malignant tumours. 7th edition. Oxford: Wiley-Blackwell; 2009.
43. Verbeke CS, Gladhaug IP. Resection margin involvement and tumour origin in pancreatic head cancer. Br J Surg 2012;99:1036–49.
44. Pomianowska E, Clausen OP, Gladhaug IP. Reclassification of tumour origin in resected periampullary adenocarcinomas reveals underrecognised diagnosis of distal bile duct cancer. Eur J Surg Oncol 2012;38:1043–50.
45. Griffin JF, Smalley SR, Jewell W, et al. Patterns of failure after curative resection of pancreatic carcinoma. Cancer 1990;66:56–61.
46. Tepper J, Nardi G, Sutt H. Carcinoma of the pancreas: review of MGH experience from 1963 to 1973: analysis of surgical failure and implications for radiation therapy. Cancer 1976;37:1519–24.
47. Westerdahl J, Andrén-Sandberg Å, Ihse I. Recurrence of exocrine pancreatic cancer: local or hepatic? Hepatogastroenterology 1993;40:384–7.
48. Kayahara M, Nagakawa T, Ueno K, et al. An evaluation of radical resection for pancreatic cancer based on the mode of recurrence as determined by autopsy and diagnostic imaging. Cancer 1983;72:2118–23.
49. Neoptolemos JP, Stocken DD, Friess H, et al, European Study Group for Pancreatic Cancer. A randomized trial of chemoradiotherapy and chemotherapy after resection of pancreatic cancer. N Engl J Med 2004;350:1200–10.
50. Ghaneh P, Neoptolemos JP. Conclusions from the European Study Group for Pancreatic Cancer adjuvant trial of chemoradiotherapy and chemotherapy for pancreatic cancer. Surg Oncol Clin N Am 2004;13:567–87, vii–viii.

51. Picozzi VJ, Pisters PW, Vickers SM, et al. Strength of the evidence: adjuvant therapy for resected pancreatic cancer. J Gastrointest Surg 2008;12:657–61.
52. Moertel CG, Frytak S, Hahn RG, et al. Gastrointestinal Tumor Study Group. Therapy of locally unresectable pancreatic carcinoma: a randomized comparison of high dose (6000 rads) radiation alone, moderate dose radiation (4000 rads + 5-fluorouracil), and high dose radiation + 5-fluorouracil. Cancer 1981;48: 1705–10.
53. Wilkowski R. Gastrointestinal Tumor Study Group. Further evidence of effective adjuvant combined radiation and chemotherapy following curative resection of pancreatic cancer. Cancer 1987;59:2006–10.
54. Hishinuma S, Ogata Y, Tomikawa M, et al. Patterns of recurrence after curative resection of pancreatic cancer, based on autopsy findings. J Gastrointest Surg 2006;10:511–8.
55. Fatima J, Schnelldorfer T, Barton J, et al. Pancreatoduodenectomy for ductal adenocarcinoma. Implications of positive margin on survival. Arch Surg 2010; 145:167–72.
56. Washington K, Berlin J, Branton P, et al. Protocol for the examination of specimens from patients with carcinoma of the exocrine pancreas. College of American Pathologists. Available at: http://www.cap.org/. Accessed February 1, 2011.

How to Define and Manage Borderline Resectable Pancreatic Cancer

Pavlos Papavasiliou, MD[a,b], Yun Shin Chun, MD[c],
John P. Hoffman, MD[c,*]

KEYWORDS

- Borderline resectable pancreatic cancer • Neoadjuvant therapy
- Surgical techniques

KEY POINTS

- The anatomic classification of borderline resectable pancreatic cancer is now more clearly defined, although complete consensus has not been reached.
- Neoadjuvant therapy allows for selection of patients who would benefit from resectional surgery and increases the likelihood of a negative resection margin.
- To achieve a negative margin of resection, surgeons should be familiar with the various techniques of venous and arterial resection.
- Pathologic response to therapy serves as the strongest prognostic indicator, as well as a guide for comparison of treatment strategies in future trials.

INTRODUCTION

Historically, borderline resectable (BLR) pancreatic cancer has had many definitions, which has made interpretation of treatment data and outcomes difficult. Advances in imaging, surgical technique, and the potential benefit of neoadjuvant therapy have emphasized the need for uniform classification, and recent efforts have produced a clearer definition. Despite these efforts, prospective randomized trials are lacking in the literature. This article reviews current definitions, treatment sequences, outcomes, and prognostic factors associated with BLR pancreatic cancer.

[a] Texas Oncology Surgical Specialists, Baylor Sammons Cancer Center, 3410 Worth Street, Suite 160, Dallas, TX 75246, USA; [b] Department of Surgery, Baylor University Medical Center, Dallas, TX, USA; [c] Department of Surgical Oncology, Fox Chase Cancer Center, 333 Cottman Avenue, Philadelphia, PA 19111, USA
* Corresponding author.
E-mail address: JP_Hoffman@fccc.edu

Surg Clin N Am 93 (2013) 663–674
http://dx.doi.org/10.1016/j.suc.2013.02.005
0039-6109/13/$ – see front matter © 2013 Elsevier Inc. All rights reserved.

DEFINITIONS
Anatomic

Borderline as an adjective describing resectability of pancreatic cancer was first used in an article by Maurer and colleagues[1] in 1999. The category of borderline resectable (BLR) pancreatic cancer has been used for tumors that are between the resectable and locally advanced categories. A definition of BLR pancreatic cancer based on multidetector computed tomography (CT) was proposed at a consensus conference sponsored by the Americas Hepato-Pancreato-Biliary Association (AHPBA), the Society for Surgery of the Alimentary Tract (SSAT) and the Society for Surgical Oncology (SSO). This definition was adopted by the National Comprehensive Cancer Network (NCCN).[2] Borderline resectability was based on tumor involvement of the superior mesenteric vein (SMV) and/or portal vein (PV), hepatic artery (HA), and superior mesenteric artery (SMA) (**Table 1**). However, the definition of the degree of venous involvement that constitutes borderline resectability varied among the consensus authors. Callery and colleagues[3] defined BLR as abutment, encasement, or reconstructible occlusion of the SMV and/or PV, whereas Abrams and colleagues[4] specified venous abutment of greater than or equal to 180° of the circumference of the SMV/PV. These definitions vary from those of the M.D. Anderson Cancer Center (**Table 2**), which defines BLR as reconstructible occlusion of the SMV-PV, whereas abutment and impingement are considered resectable.[5,6] It has been well documented that patients with SMV/PV abutment alone, without deformity of the vessel, have a significantly better prognosis than those with increasing degrees of impingement.[7–9] Therefore, any series in the future using this definition of BLR will by definition have better outcomes regardless of treatment type. To further complicate matters, the NCCN has recently changed its BLR definition to exclude abutment of the veins (Version I.2013).

Similarly, the degree of arterial involvement that constitutes borderline resectability is under debate. Whereas the M.D. Anderson definition of BLR includes encasement (>180°) of the hepatic artery and abutment (≤180°) of the SMA and/or celiac axis, the NCCN specifies no extension to the celiac axis and less than or equal to 180° abutment of the HA in their definition of BLR. Data to support or reject these definitions are lacking. Regarding involvement of the HA or celiac axis, there are too few cases in the literature to make any conclusions, other than there is a high likelihood of leaving positive margins and hospital stay is prolonged after resection (**Table 3** for discrepancies in anatomic definition).

Table 1	
NCCN guideline criteria for anatomic definition of BLR pancreatic cancer*	
Vessel	**Degree of Involvement**
SMV/PV	Impingement and narrowing of the lumen*
	Encasement without encasement of nearby arteries
	Short-segment venous occlusion due to thrombus or encasement with suitable vessel proximal and distal allowing for resection and reconstruction
Gastroduodenal artery (GDA)/HA	GDA encasement up to hepatic artery with either short segment encasement or direct abutment of hepatic artery, without celiac axis extension
SMA	Abutment not to exceed 180° of the vessel wall

* NCCN Version I.2013.

Table 2
M.D. Anderson system for classifying patients with BLR pancreatic cancer

A	Abutment of SMA or celiac axis ≤180°, abutment or encasement short segment HA, short-segment occlusion of SMV, PV, or SMV-PV confluence amenable to resection and reconstruction
B	Known lymph node involvement or concern for metastatic disease
C	Comorbid conditions requiring workup and evaluation before surgery, marginal performance status expected eventually to improve

Until the definition of BLR can be standardized, reporting should specify not only what definitions are used but also which of the specific categories (SMV abutment impingement or occlusion, SMA or HA abutment, and by how many degrees) define the resectability status of each of the patients being reported. The relative values of different neoadjuvant and adjuvant programs will remain uncertain until the resectability status of patients is strictly defined. These data should be collected and reported to eventually arrive at a true consensus definition of BLR. Until such time, the BLR categories can be separated into major and minor, the former being essentially the M.D. Anderson definition and the latter including the various abutments and impingements without occlusion of the SMV/PV. The intent of resectability status is to stage patients by means of imaging, such that the results of their treatments can be compared. It is futile to argue whether one or another definition is correct, but it is crucial to clearly define the imaging characteristics of the treated group being reported to correctly assess the relative value of the treatment regimen.

Nonanatomic

The M.D. Anderson group has proposed 3 categories of BLR patients, including 2 groups based on nonimaging criteria. Patients in group A are BLR based on vascular involvement, as outlined in **Table 2**. Patients in group B have findings suggestive of but not diagnostic for distant metastases, including suspicious CT findings or known lymph node metastases. Patients in group C have a marginal performance status or severe comorbidities precluding immediate operation, but potentially improving such that they could have surgery in the future.

IMAGING

Advances in CT imaging have made a more precise classification of BLR pancreatic cancer possible. Arterial and venous phase contrast, multiplanar, three-dimensional CT can help delineate the extent of tumor involvement of the vasculature, and assist

Table 3
Discrepancies in imaging definitions of BLR

Vessel Involvement	M.D. Anderson	Callery/Abrams (Consensus)	NCCN I.2013
SMV/PV	Short-segment occlusion amenable to resection and reconstruction	Abutment with or without impingement/ encasement	Distortion, narrowing or reconstructible occlusion
SMA/HA	≤180° abutment of celiac axis or SMA, abutment or encasement of HA	<180° SMA abutment; involvement of HA amenable to Reconstruction	<180° abutment SMA, abutment or short segment encasement of HA

in preoperative planning for vascular reconstruction. Compared with magnetic resonance imaging (MRI), both modalities are equal in assessing lymphadenopathy, liver metastases, vascular involvement, and unresectability. It is our preference to use CT as our imaging modality as it is most familiar to surgeons (**Fig. 1**). Although CT is only modestly helpful in measuring response to treatment (response generally results in replacement of cancer cells by fibrosis rather than shrinkage), interpreting resectability based on vascular involvement can also prove challenging, particularly in patients who have undergone treatment with radiation therapy.[10] It is the authors' practice to rely more on the pretreatment study, the posttreatment carbohydrate antigen (CA)19-9, and the frozen sections during surgery to determine the extent of resection after neoadjuvant therapy should the posttreatment CT or MRI prove to be equivocal. The most challenging situation is when the radiologist mentions "dirty fat" near the arteries, as this often is the result of changes in the soft tissue from the radiotherapy, and not from cancer extension (**Fig. 2**).

Endoscopic ultrasonography (EUS) is accurate in assessing vascular involvement, although its role is typically reserved for obtaining a tissue diagnosis via fine-needle aspiration (FNA) before initiating neoadjuvant therapy. The sensitivity, specificity, and accuracy of obtaining a diagnosis of pancreatic cancer from EUS-FNA vary from 75% to 90%, 82% to 100%, and 85%, respectively.[11] Endoscopic retrograde cholangiopancreatography at the time of EUS allows for common bile duct stent placement for obstructing cancers.

NEOADJUVANT THERAPY FOR BLR PANCREATIC CANCER

The overall goals in the treatment of BLR pancreatic cancer are to achieve a negative margin of resection, guarantee that the patient will receive adjuvant therapy, and select those with systemic disease who would not benefit from resection. No phase III trial between neoadjuvant and postoperative adjuvant therapy has been performed, but there are many retrospective comparisons using the BLR criteria that favor neoadjuvant therapy for these cancers that almost certainly would have had a positive resection margin if surgery were performed first (**Table 4**).

The rationale for neoadjuvant treatment in BLR pancreatic cancer includes the following:

1. Most patients already have microscopic metastases at the time of diagnosis.[12,13] Providing an observation period during neoadjuvant treatment allows the discovery of initially occult metastases and thus unnecessary surgery is avoided.

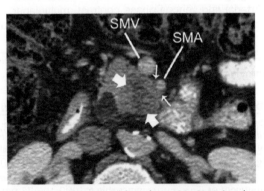

Fig. 1. BLR tumor with SMV abutment and less than 180° SMA involvement. Large arrows indicate the cancer, small arrows the SMA and SMV abutments.

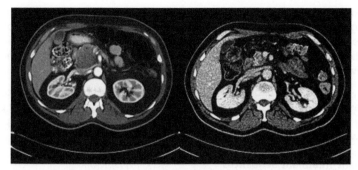

Fig. 2. Downstaging by imaging. This patient received neoadjuvant gemcitabine-based chemoradiation followed by resection. CA 19-9 levels dropped from 3940 to 10 before and after neoadjuvant therapy. CT images show bilateral narrowing of the PV before treatment (Ishikawa IV) with improvement in narrowing after treatment. This patient showed a complete pathologic response to therapy after resection.

2. It provides assurance that all patients receive radiation and chemotherapy, as up to 20% of those undergoing initial surgery do not receive adjuvant therapy because of postoperative complications, poor recovery, or metastases.[14]
3. Retrospective comparisons have shown that the percentage of positive margin resections is much less after preoperative therapy in these BLR cancers.[15]

Table 4
Studies using the definition of BLR pancreatic cancer

Study	Treatment Sequence	Number of Patients	Definition Used in Study	Median Overall Survival of Patients Who Completed All Therapy (Mo)
Katz et al,[17,29] 2008	Chemotherapy, followed by chemoradiation, followed by surgery	160	M.D. Anderson	40
Brown et al,[21] 2008	Chemoradiation, then chemotherapy	13	AHPBA/Callery	Not reached
Stokes et al,[18] 2011	Chemoradiation	40	M.D. Anderson	12
Sahora et al,[19,20] 2011	Chemotherapy	33	AHPBA[a]	22
Patel et al,[36] 2011	Chemotherapy followed by intensity modulated radiation therapy	17	AHPBA/Callery	16
Barugola et al,[37] 2012	Upfront resection, preoperative chemotherapy, and preoperative chemoradiation	41	AHPBA/Callery	35

[a] AHPBA criteria not specified in study, and definition applied retrospectively.

4. Smaller radiation fields target the tumor and surrounding tissue to be resected, sparing more surrounding normal tissue compared with postoperative radiotherapy.
5. The treatment effect can be examined and quantified histopathologically.
6. Radiation therapy is delivered to better oxygenated tumor cells, and is thus more effective.

Overall, the benefit of neoadjuvant therapy is best described by Papalezova and colleagues[16]: "the primary effect of preoperative chemoradiation is to select patients who are most likely to benefit from resection and that this is not at the expense of patients who do not undergo resection."

Neoadjuvant Treatment Sequences

There are differences in opinion regarding treatment sequencing with regard to when and if radiation treatment should be applied. No randomized comparisons have been done.

Chemotherapy followed by chemoradiation followed by surgery

The argument for this sequence is that immediate systemic treatment is given to patients with occult micrometastases. Chemoradiation for optimal local control is administered only to those patients who have not progressed with systemic disease. In addition, initial treatment with radiation therapy can lead to marrow suppression, which limits the ability to receive adequate amounts of future chemotherapy.

The M.D. Anderson series from Katz and colleagues[17] used this treatment sequence. Chemotherapy (gemcitabine alone or in combination) was used for 2 to 4 months, followed by chemoradiotherapy (5-fluorouracil, paclitaxel, gemcitabine or capecitabine at radiosensitizing doses). One hundred and sixty patients were classified as BLR over a period of 7 years. Forty-one percent of patients completed neoadjuvant treatment and went on to resection. Most patients who did not make it to resection did so because of progression of either local or distant cancer during or after completion of neoadjuvant therapy. The overall R1 resection rate from this study was 6%, and no patients underwent an R2 resection. Median overall survival for the entire group was 18 months, with a 5-year survival rate of 18% for all patients. Of the patients who underwent resection, median overall survival was 40 months, with a 5-year survival rate of 36%. Disease-free survival was 24 months for patients who underwent resection; 59% of patients had a recurrence within a median of 25 months (range 2–88 months) among those who were alive at the time of the report.

Chemoradiation followed by surgery

This was the method of treatment from the earliest development of neoadjuvant therapy in the 1980s. The rationale for this sequence is an optimal local tumor effect with a relatively short interval to surgical resection. The chemotherapy is given primarily to enhance the radiation effects. Stokes and colleagues[18] published results from a prospective protocol using capecitabine-based chemoradiation, followed by surgery. Thirty-four patients with BLR pancreatic cancer underwent neoadjuvant chemoradiation and were restaged. Seventy-three percent of these patients went on to successful resection. Median overall survival from date of diagnosis for all patients classified as BLR was 12 months, and median overall survival for patients who underwent resection was 23 months. Two patients had an R1 resection (both arterial margins), and there were no R2 resections. Eighty-eight percent of the patients who underwent resection received postresectional adjuvant chemotherapy. All of the BLR patients were defined by the M.D. Anderson scheme, and thus they either had SMV/PV occlusion or SMA or HA abutment. The end results are similar to the M. D. Anderson series of Katz and colleagues.[17] The resectability for the 40 patients with BLR cancers was 40% and the median survival for those with resection was 23 months.

Chemotherapy followed by surgery

Sahora and colleagues[19,20] published results from 2 prospective phase II trials in which the classification as BLR pancreatic cancer was applied retrospectively. The treatment plan consisted of a gemcitabine/oxaliplatin regimen for the first trial and a gemcitabine/docetaxel combination in the second, with restaging at the completion of treatment. Of the 15 patients in the first study who were classified retrospectively as BLR, 10 patients had abutment or encasement of the SMV or PV, and 5 had additional or exclusive short-segment abutment of the SMA. Seven of the 15 patients initially classified as BLR underwent resection, although their outcomes were not reported. Of the 12 patients in the second study with BLR cancers treated by gemcitabine and docetaxel (retrospectively characterized), 4 underwent resection. This study included patients considered initially to have unresectable disease, and overall, 8 of these patients underwent resection. Four of the 8 with resections developed local recurrences, despite an R0 resection rate of 87%, perhaps related to the deletion of radiation therapy.

Chemoradiation followed by prolonged chemotherapy

The series reported by Brown and colleagues[21] used prolonged chemotherapy (mostly gemcitabine-based regimens) after chemoradiotherapy when patients were either too weak for surgery or imaging continued to show involved vascular margins. The chemotherapy was given for a median of 3 cycles after completion of chemoradiotherapy. Histopathologic response, quantified as percent fibrosis score (100% equals a complete pathologic response), was associated with improved overall and disease-free survival. A potential advantage of the chemoradiation followed by chemotherapy approach is that a longer interval between radiation and surgery provides for a continued cytotoxic treatment effect of radiation with time, analogous to emerging data on rectal cancer.[22]

It is hoped that future trials will assess the relative values of these approaches to neoadjuvant therapy for BLR patients. Currently, several individual trials are underway using newer chemotherapeutic and radiotherapeutic regimens, but none are comparing these different approaches.

SURGERY FOR BLR PANCREATIC CANCER

Achieving an R0 resection can be challenging in patients with BLR pancreatic cancer. The ability to resect and reconstruct vascular structures is essential when treating patients who have been deemed resectable after neoadjuvant therapy. However, the accuracy of imaging is particularly poor for vascular involvement after neoadjuvant therapy. False-positive results are common.[10] The sensitivity of CT/MRI for detecting vascular involvement after neoadjuvant chemoradiation is 71% and the specificity is 58%. In addition, the radiographic response does not predict resectability.[23] Approaches to the various vascular involvements are discussed in the following sections.

Preoperative Planning

After neoadjuvant treatment, cross-sectional imaging to determine the extent of vascular involvement can be misleading. Therefore, plans for vascular resection and reconstruction should be based on pretherapy imaging. High-quality CT imaging provides details of tumor involvement and anatomic variation that play a crucial role in obtaining an R0 resection with low morbidity.

Vein Involvement

Resection and reconstruction of the SMV or PV at high-volume centers has been shown to be associated with a low rate of perioperative morbidity and similar R0 resection rates compared with patients who have undergone standard pancreatoduodenectomy performed without venous resection.[24,25] Detailed anatomic information on the PV, SMV, and its first-order branches can be obtained with triphasic, multiplanar CT imaging.[26–28] The approach to reconstruction is based on the location of tumor involvement of the SMV in relation to the jejunal and ileal branches.

Reconstruction of the SMV/PV can take many forms. Tangential resection for partial involvement can be performed either with primary closure or vein patch reconstruction. When performing primary closure, it is helpful to clamp the vein transversely above and below the involved portion of vein to allow for longitudinal closure. Patch reconstruction is typically done using the greater saphenous vein.

Tumor involvement of the jejunal or ileal branches of the SMV can pose a challenge because of the variability in anatomy.[29,30] The jejunal branch of the SMV courses anterior to the SMA in up to 41% of patients, which typically allows for less challenging dissection of the SMV and its branches.[31] However, the more typical posterior course of the first jejunal branch renders dissection more difficult and the likelihood of SMA injury during attempts to control venous bleeding is higher. This anatomic relationship is easily assessed on preoperative CT imaging, and should be known before pancreatoduodenectomy.

Segmental resection of the SMV can be reconstructed with an interposition vein graft using the internal jugular or superficial femoral vein. Either the jejunal or ileal branch can be ligated, provided that sufficient vein diameter remains (at least the diameter of the SMA). Katz and colleagues[29,30] have described reconstruction of the confluence of the jejunal and ileal branches by ligating the jejunal branch and reconstructing the ileal branch. It is the authors' preference to involve vascular surgery in the reconstruction process.

Arterial Involvement

HA reconstruction can typically be accomplished using a polytetrafluoroethylene interposition graft or the saphenous vein. Partial arterial wall resection with vein patch reconstruction is another option if encasement is not present (**Fig. 3**). Abutment of the SMA is generally handled with fine dissection, preferably including the adventitia of the artery. SMA encasement or abutment for more than 180° is considered unresectable, precluding reconstruction.[32] However, cases with debatable SMA involvement, particularly after neoadjuvant chemoradiotherapy and displaying "dirty fat," should be explored with the intention of resection unless obvious arterial wall involvement is seen.

PROGNOSTIC FACTORS IN BLR PANCREATIC CANCER
Degree of Venous Involvement

In 1992, Ishikawa and colleagues[9] proposed a classification system for the degree of PV/SMV involvement based on preoperative angiography. The degree of venous involvement was classified into 5 categories: (I) normal SMV contour; (II) smooth shift without narrowing; (III) unilateral narrowing; (IV) bilateral narrowing; (V) bilateral narrowing with collateral veins visible (**Table 5**). This study found a 3-year survival rate of 59% for patients classified as having I to III vein involvement. Patients classified as IV or V showed a worse survival than patients deemed unresectable.

A more recent study by Chun and colleagues[8] from Fox Chase Cancer Center classified 109 patients with BLR pancreatic cancer according to the Ishikawa system.

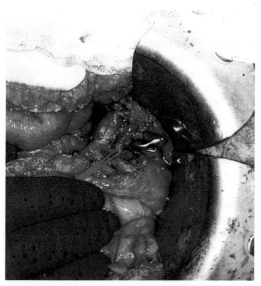

Fig. 3. Greater saphenous vein patch reconstruction of the HA.

Sixty-eight percent of these patients received preoperative chemoradiation, and 41% underwent venous resection. Overall, preoperative therapy was found to correlate with higher rates of R0 resection, negative lymph nodes, smaller tumors measured after resection, and improved overall survival.

For patients with unilateral narrowing (Ishikawa types II/III), neoadjuvant chemoradiation improved R0 resection rates (71% R0 resection rate with neoadjuvant chemoradiation vs 5% R0 resection without neoadjuvant chemoradiation) and overall survival (26 months vs 10 months). Patients with bilateral narrowing or occlusion showed no difference in R0 resection rates or overall survival whether they received neoadjuvant chemoradiation or not, although the numbers for comparison were small and there were no patients classified as Ishikawa V in the group who underwent surgery first. Therefore, neoadjuvant therapy is recommended for these patients unless data emerge that show equivalence in outcome for initial surgery.

Pathologic Response

As neoadjuvant treatment for all cancers becomes more prevalent, so does the finding that response to treatment is a major prognostic indicator. For pancreatic cancer, there have been differences reported in how to quantify response to treatment.

Table 5
Ishikawa grading system to define degree of venous involvement

Ishikawa Grade	Venous Involvement
I	Normal contour
II	Smooth shift
III	Unilateral narrowing
IV	Bilateral narrowing
V	Bilateral narrowing with collateral vein

Chatterjee and colleagues[33] reported results using classification systems based on the percentage of residual tumor remaining (Evans classification) and the ratio of residual tumor cells and stroma (College of American Pathologists). Of the patients who had a complete response to treatment (n = 6), none developed recurrence or died of disease during follow-up. Patients were analyzed in 2 groups: (1) complete response or less than 5% viable tumor and (2) patients with 5% or more viable tumor. Patients with complete response or less than 5% viable tumor had improved overall and disease-free survival, and none had a positive margin of resection (vs 13% positive margins of resection for all others).

Chun and colleagues[34] reported outcomes based on response to neoadjuvant chemoradiation using a classification system based on mean percent fibrosis. On all the histologic slides from the resected specimens, the areas of fibrosis were outlined and the percentage of cancer cells within those areas of fibrosis were determined. The results from each of the slides were summed and then averaged. Patients with a major response, classified as greater than 95% fibrosis, had a 66-month median overall survival and a 5-year survival rate of 53%. On multivariate analysis, major response was the only independent factor that correlated with overall survival. Major response also correlated with R0 resection rate, negative lymph nodes, and smaller pathologic tumor size (although the tumors were equal or greater in size at first diagnosis).

These results suggest that identifying ways of increasing the likelihood of achieving a complete or near complete pathologic response will have the biggest impact on outcome in future trials. More investigation is needed to determine which variables before surgery predict major pathologic responses and to identify systemic and local therapies that improve pathologic responses. So far, CA19-9 reversion to normal levels and partial response as measured by RECIST criteria (Response Evaluation Criteria In Solid Tumors) by imaging are the best known surrogates for tissue response, but neither is definitive.[34,35]

SUMMARY

BLR pancreatic cancer presents many challenges with regard to definition, best systemic and local therapy, surgical approach, and interpretation of outcomes data. Further clarification and consensus on the definition of BLR pancreatic cancer will allow for further data collection and cooperation in future efforts to make progress and standardize treatment. There are currently several phase II trials of neoadjuvant treatments (chemoradiation ± chemotherapy or chemotherapy alone) including some or all of these BLR patients. It is hoped that imaging characteristics and other parameters of BLR status will be clear enough to allow for true progress in therapy for these patients.

REFERENCES

1. Maurer CA, Zgraggen K, Buchler MW. Pancreatic carcinoma. Optimizing therapy by adjuvant and neoadjuvant therapy? Zentralbl Chir 1999;124(5):401–7 [in German].
2. Tempero MA, Behrman S, Ben-Josef E, et al. Pancreatic adenocarcinoma: Clinical Practice Guidelines in Oncology. J Natl Compr Canc Netw 2005;3(5):598–626.
3. Callery MP, Chang KJ, Fishman EK, et al. Pretreatment assessment of resectable and borderline resectable pancreatic cancer: expert consensus statement. Ann Surg Oncol 2009;16(7):1727–33.
4. Abrams RA, Lowy AM, O'Reilly EM, et al. Combined modality treatment of resectable and borderline resectable pancreas cancer: expert consensus statement. Ann Surg Oncol 2009;16(7):1751–6.

5. Varadhachary GR, Tamm EP, Crane C, et al. Borderline resectable pancreatic cancer. Curr Treat Options Gastroenterol 2005;8(5):377–84.
6. Varadhachary GR, Tamm EP, Abbruzzese JL, et al. Borderline resectable pancreatic cancer: definitions, management, and role of preoperative therapy. Ann Surg Oncol 2006;13(8):1035–46.
7. Fukuda S, Oussoultzoglou E, Bachellier P, et al. Significance of the depth of portal vein wall invasion after curative resection for pancreatic adenocarcinoma. Arch Surg 2007;142(2):172–9 [discussion: 180].
8. Chun YS, Milestone BN, Watson JC, et al. Defining venous involvement in borderline resectable pancreatic cancer. Ann Surg Oncol 2010;17(11): 2832–8.
9. Ishikawa O, Ohigashi H, Imaoka S, et al. Preoperative indications for extended pancreatectomy for locally advanced pancreas cancer involving the portal vein. Ann Surg 1992;215(3):231–6.
10. Katz MH, Fleming JB, Bhosale P, et al. Response of borderline resectable pancreatic cancer to neoadjuvant therapy is not reflected by radiographic indicators. Cancer 2012;118:5749–56.
11. Boujaoude J. Role of endoscopic ultrasound in diagnosis and therapy of pancreatic adenocarcinoma. World J Gastroenterol 2007;13(27):3662–6.
12. Haeno H, Gonen M, Davis MB, et al. Computational modeling of pancreatic cancer reveals kinetics of metastasis suggesting optimum treatment strategies. Cell 2012;148(1–2):362–75.
13. Rhim AD, Mirek ET, Aiello NM, et al. EMT and dissemination precede pancreatic tumor formation. Cell 2012;148(1–2):349–61.
14. Sohn TA, Yeo CJ, Cameron JL, et al. Resected adenocarcinoma of the pancreas-616 patients: results, outcomes, and prognostic indicators. J Gastrointest Surg 2000;4(6):567–79.
15. Pingpank JF, Hoffman JP, Ross EA, et al. Effect of preoperative chemoradiotherapy on surgical margin status of resected adenocarcinoma of the head of the pancreas. J Gastrointest Surg 2001;5(2):121–30.
16. Papalezova KT, Tyler DS, Blazer DG 3rd, et al. Does preoperative therapy optimize outcomes in patients with resectable pancreatic cancer? J Surg Oncol 2012; 106(1):111–8.
17. Katz MH, Pisters PW, Evans DB, et al. Borderline resectable pancreatic cancer: the importance of this emerging stage of disease. J Am Coll Surg 2008;206(5): 833–46 [discussion: 846–8].
18. Stokes JB, Nolan NJ, Stelow EB, et al. Preoperative capecitabine and concurrent radiation for borderline resectable pancreatic cancer. Ann Surg Oncol 2011; 18(3):619–27.
19. Sahora K, Kuehrer I, Eisenhut A, et al. NeoGemOx: gemcitabine and oxaliplatin as neoadjuvant treatment for locally advanced, nonmetastasized pancreatic cancer. Surgery 2011;149(3):311–20.
20. Sahora K, Kuehrer I, Schindl M, et al. NeoGemTax: gemcitabine and docetaxel as neoadjuvant treatment for locally advanced nonmetastasized pancreatic cancer. World J Surg 2011;35(7):1580–9.
21. Brown KM, Siripurapu V, Davidson M, et al. Chemoradiation followed by chemotherapy before resection for borderline pancreatic adenocarcinoma. Am J Surg 2008;195(3):318–21.
22. Kalady MF, de Campos-Lobato LF, Stocchi L, et al. Predictive factors of pathologic complete response after neoadjuvant chemoradiation for rectal cancer. Ann Surg 2009;250(4):582–9.

23. Donahue TR, Isacoff WH, Hines OJ, et al. Downstaging chemotherapy and alteration in the classic computed tomography/magnetic resonance imaging signs of vascular involvement in patients with pancreaticobiliary malignant tumors: influence on patient selection for surgery. Arch Surg 2011;146(7):836–43.

24. Tseng JF, Raut CP, Lee JE, et al. Pancreaticoduodenectomy with vascular resection: margin status and survival duration. J Gastrointest Surg 2004;8(8):935–49 [discussion: 949–50].

25. Raut CP, Tseng JF, Sun CC, et al. Impact of resection status on pattern of failure and survival after pancreaticoduodenectomy for pancreatic adenocarcinoma. Ann Surg 2007;246(1):52–60.

26. Graf O, Boland GW, Kaufman JA, et al. Anatomic variants of mesenteric veins: depiction with helical CT venography. AJR Am J Roentgenol 1997;168(5):1209–13.

27. Ito K, Blasbalg R, Hussain SM, et al. Portal vein and its tributaries: evaluation with thin-section three-dimensional contrast-enhanced dynamic fat-suppressed MR imaging. Radiology 2000;215(2):381–6.

28. Kim HJ, Ko YT, Lim JW, et al. Radiologic anatomy of the superior mesenteric vein and branching patterns of the first jejunal trunk: evaluation using multi-detector row CT venography. Surg Radiol Anat 2007;29(1):67–75.

29. Katz MH, Fleming JB, Pisters PW, et al. Anatomy of the superior mesenteric vein with special reference to the surgical management of first-order branch involvement at pancreaticoduodenectomy. Ann Surg 2008;248(6):1098–102.

30. Katz MH, Lee JE, Pisters PW, et al. Retroperitoneal dissection in patients with borderline resectable pancreatic cancer: operative principles and techniques. J Am Coll Surg 2012;215(2):e11–8.

31. Papavasiliou P, Arrangoiz R, Zhu F, et al. The anatomic course of the first jejunal branch of the superior mesenteric vein in relation to the superior mesenteric artery. Int J Surg Oncol 2012;2012:538769.

32. Stitzenberg KB, Watson JC, Roberts A, et al. Survival after pancreatectomy with major arterial resection and reconstruction. Ann Surg Oncol 2008;15(5): 1399–406.

33. Chatterjee D, Katz MH, Rashid A, et al. Histologic grading of the extent of residual carcinoma following neoadjuvant chemoradiation in pancreatic ductal adenocarcinoma: a predictor for patient outcome. Cancer 2012;118(12):3182–90.

34. Chun YS, Cooper HS, Cohen SJ, et al. Significance of pathologic response to preoperative therapy in pancreatic cancer. Ann Surg Oncol 2011;18(13):3601–7.

35. Katz MH, Varadhachary GR, Fleming JB, et al. Serum CA 19-9 as a marker of resectability and survival in patients with potentially resectable pancreatic cancer treated with neoadjuvant chemoradiation. Ann Surg Oncol 2010;17(7):1794–801.

36. Patel M, Hoffe S, Malafa M, et al. Neoadjuvant GTX chemotherapy and IMRT-based chemoradiation for borderline resectable pancreatic cancer. J Surg Oncology 2011;104:155–61.

37. Barugola G, Partelli S, Crippa S, et al. Outcomes after resection of locally advanced or borderline resectable pancreatic cancer after neoadjuvant therapy. Am J Surgery 2012;203:132–9.

Management of Pancreatic Neuroendocrine Tumors

Paxton V. Dickson, MD, Stephen W. Behrman, MD*

KEYWORDS

- Pancreatic neuroendocrine tumors • Surgery • Metastatic neuroendocrine tumors
- Chemotherapy • Targeted therapy

KEY POINTS

- Pancreatic neuroendocrine tumors account for 1% to 2% of pancreatic neoplasms and may occur sporadically or as part of a hereditary syndrome.
- Patients may present with symptoms related to hormone secretion by functional tumors or with symptoms related to locally advanced or metastatic nonfunctional tumors.
- An increasing number of asymptomatic pancreatic neuroendocrine tumors are detected incidentally during abdominal imaging performed for other reasons.
- The management of localized pancreatic neuroendocrine tumors is surgical resection.
- Hepatic metastases are common and their management involves a variety of liver-directed therapies, which should be tailored according to extent of disease, symptoms, presence of extrahepatic metastases, and patient performance status.

INTRODUCTION

Pancreatic neuroendocrine tumors (PNETs) constitute 1% to 2% of pancreatic neoplasms and show unique genetics, biology, and prognosis relative to pancreatic adenocarcinomas.[1–3] Furthermore, although PNETs share similar histologic features with neuroendocrine tumors from other sites (ie, midgut carcinoids), it has become increasingly apparent that they differ in molecular pathogenesis, clinical behavior, and response to certain therapies.[4,5] PNETs comprise a diverse group of neoplasms including functional and nonfunctional tumors as well as tumors that may represent a manifestation of a hereditary neuroendocrine syndrome. The heterogeneity in the clinical presentation of PNETs creates unique challenges in their management. Moreover, most patients present with regionally advanced or metastatic disease[6] (groups for which no definitive treatment algorithms exist). This review addresses the clinical

Division of Surgical Oncology, Department of Surgery, University of Tennessee Health Science Center, 910 Madison Avenue, Suite 208, Memphis, TN 38163, USA
* Corresponding author.
E-mail address: sbehrman@uthsc.edu

Surg Clin N Am 93 (2013) 675–691
http://dx.doi.org/10.1016/j.suc.2013.02.001
0039-6109/13/$ – see front matter © 2013 Elsevier Inc. All rights reserved.

surgical.theclinics.com

presentation and evaluation of patients with PNETs as well as surgical and nonsurgical strategies available for the treatment of these patients.

CLINICAL PRESENTATION

PNETs are classified as either functional or nonfunctional, depending on whether a patient experiences symptoms related to excess hormone production by the tumor. Although less common, functional tumors account for a fascinating spectrum of clinical syndromes resulting from hypersecretion of hormones such as gastrin, insulin, glucagon, vasoactive intestinal peptide, and rarely somatostatin.[7,8] A detailed description of the diagnostic criteria and clinical manifestations (**Table 1**) of these functional tumors is beyond the scope of this article; however, it is important for the

Table 1
Functional PNETs

Tumor	Hormone	Clinical Presentation	Diagnostic Criteria
Insulinoma	Insulin	Hypoglycemia, resulting in intermittent confusion, weakness, diaphoresis, nausea; symptoms often relieved by eating	72 h fast: plasma glucose <45 mg/dL; insulin ≥6 μU/mL; insulin/glucose ratio >0.3; C-peptide level ≥0.2 nmol/L; proinsulin level ≥5 pmol/L; absence of sulfonylurea
Gastrinoma	Gastrin	Acid hypersecretion resulting in refractory PUD, abdominal pain, and diarrhea (Zollinger-Ellison syndrome)	Increased fasting serum gastrin level off PPIs in the setting of gastric pH <2.5; secretin stimulation test with paradoxic increase in serum gastrin by ≥200 pg/mL
VIPoma	Vasoactive intestinal peptide	Profound secretory diarrhea, electrolyte disturbances (watery diarrhea, hypokalemia, achlorhydria syndrome)	Unexplained high-volume watery diarrhea and serum VIP level >75 pg/mL
Glucagonoma	Glucagon	NME, glucose intolerance, cachexia, deep vein thrombosis	Markedly increased fasting serum glucagon level (>500 pg/mL); patients typically present with NME
Somatostatinoma	Somatostatin	Diabetes, steatorrhea, cholelithiasis	Fasting serum somatostatin level >160 pg/mL in setting of pancreatic or duodenal mass or classic clinical signs/symptoms

Abbreviations: NME, necrotizing migratory erythema; PPIs, proton-pump inhibitors; PUD, peptic ulcer disease; VIP, vasoactive intestinal peptide.

surgeon involved in the management of these patients to be aware of their presentation, localization, and management.

Because they are not associated with a clinical syndrome, nonfunctional PNETs typically present with nonspecific symptoms such as abdominal pain, weight loss, or early satiety, and are locally advanced or metastatic at the time of diagnosis in greater than 50% of cases.[7–10] In contradistinction to adenocarcinoma, PNETs located in the pancreatic head rarely present with jaundice. Given the widespread application of high-quality cross-sectional imaging, clinicians are likely to be increasingly faced with the management of asymptomatic, incidentally found PNETs in patients undergoing abdominal imaging for other reasons.

Despite the lack of a hormonally mediated syndrome, nonfunctional PNETs often secrete several measurable peptides such as chromogranin A (CgA), neuron-specific enolase, and pancreatic polypeptide. Serum CgA is considered the best biomarker during evaluation and surveillance of patients with neuroendocrine tumors. It shows a relatively high sensitivity and specificity, and plasma levels have been shown to correlate with tumor burden, making it a useful surrogate in monitoring response to therapy.[11–13] However, CgA can be increased in patients on proton-pump inhibitors, patients with atrophic gastritis, and in patients with hepatic or renal insufficiency. Although not recommended for purposes of screening, baseline and serial serum CgA levels should be obtained at the time of PNET diagnosis and after both surgical or nonsurgical therapeutic interventions.

Although most PNETs occur as sporadic neoplasms, they may occasionally arise as manifestation of a hereditary syndrome. Multiple endocrine neoplasia type 1 (MEN1) (Wermer syndrome), von Hippel-Lindau (VHL) disease, neurofibromatosis type 1 (NF1) (von Recklinghausen disease), and tuberous sclerosis each have a well-established association with PNETs (**Table 2**).[14] When evaluating patients diagnosed with PNET, query for a family history of PNETs and other neoplasms associated with these syndromes is important.

IMAGING EVALUATION FOR PNETS

Imaging of patients with PNETs is necessary to assess local extent of the primary tumor and evaluate for regional and distant metastases. A variety of imaging modalities have been used in the initial assessment and surveillance of patients with PNETs and selection of appropriate studies is important in treatment planning.

Table 2
Hereditary neuroendocrine syndromes associated with PNETs

Hereditary Syndrome	Associated Conditions	Genetic Mutation
MEN1	Primary hyperparathyroidism, pituitary adenomas, PNETs (80%)	*MEN1* gene 11q13
VHL disease	Central nervous system vascular tumors, renal cell carcinoma, pheochromocytoma, pancreatic cystadenomas, PNETs (10%–20%)	VHL gene 3p25
Tuberous sclerosis complex	Multifocal hamartomas, debilitating neurologic deficits, PNETs (1%–2%)	TSC1 gene 9q34 TSC2 gene 16p13
NF1	Café au lait spots, superficial and deep neurofibromas, Lisch nodules, pheochromocytoma, PNETs (<5%)	NF1 gene 17q11

Cross-sectional imaging with high-quality contrast-enhanced computed tomography (CT) with dedicated pancreas protocol or magnetic resonance imaging (MRI) should be obtained and is very sensitive in detecting lesions 1 cm or greater.[15] PNETs typically appear hypervascular (**Fig. 1**), although they may occasionally have a cystic appearance or calcifications. In addition to CT or MRI, endoscopic ultrasonography (EUS) is often performed in the evaluation of patients with pancreatic neoplasms. EUS allows detection of smaller lesions[16] and may also yield more detailed assessment of the relationship of intrapancreatic tumors to pertinent ductal and vascular structures and provide improved evaluation of regional lymph nodes. Furthermore, EUS-guided fine-needle aspiration can be used to obtain a diagnosis before a definitive treatment plan is initiated.

With the exception of benign insulinomas, most PNETs overexpress somatostatin receptors; therefore, somatostatin receptor scintigraphy (SRS) is a useful modality for the detection of both primary and metastatic lesions.[17,18] Baseline whole-body SRS combined with CT (single-photon emission CT imaging) (**Fig. 2**) should be considered at the time of diagnosis to rule out occult metastases or better characterize indeterminate lesions seen on CT or MRI.[8] Given improvements in detection with current cross-sectional imaging techniques, EUS, and SRS, selective intra-arterial calcium injection with hepatic vein sampling is now rarely used to localize functional tumors. Nevertheless, familiarity with these techniques should not be abandoned, because they are still occasionally required to localize small insulinomas or gastrinomas not detected by standard imaging.

STAGING AND PATHOLOGIC CLASSIFICATION

The World Health Organization,[19] European Neuroendocrine Tumor Society,[20] and the American Joint Committee on Cancer (AJCC)[3] have proposed formal staging systems for PNETs. Although establishment of a single uniform system is unlikely, overlap within these schemas permits collection of pertinent tumor data that can be used in collaborative research efforts. The AJCC staging manual did not incorporate staging criteria for PNETs until the recent seventh edition, published in 2010. This update was based, in part, on a National Cancer Database (NCDB) analysis by Bilimoria

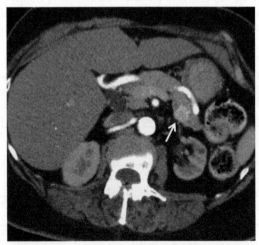

Fig. 1. PNET within the tail of the pancreas (*arrow*). These neoplasms are usually hyperintense during the arterial phase.

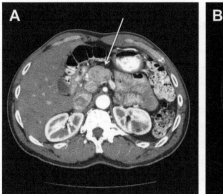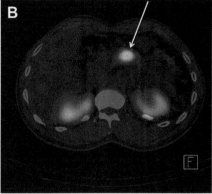

Fig. 2. SRS can be used to localize and confirm PNETs and evaluate for distant metastases. Isointense lesion is shown in the neck of the pancreas on CT (*A*), which on SRS (*B*) is confirmed to be a neuroendocrine tumor. The lesion in the neck of the pancreas is shown by the arrow in both panels.

and colleagues,[21] which reported significant survival discrimination in patients with PNET in whom AJCC sixth edition staging criteria for pancreatic adenocarcinoma were applied. The survival data from this report correlate with recent SEER (Surveillance Epidemiology and End Results)-based analyses, and collectively these studies provide robust prognostic data.[6,22] The AJCC staging criteria for PNETs and stage-specific survival data are shown in **Table 3**.

In addition to standard TNM criteria, tumor grade and differentiation have important prognostic and treatment-related implications for patients with neuroendocrine tumors.[23,24] After a diagnosis of PNET, formal assessment of these histopathologic features should be obtained. In general, neuroendocrine tumors are reported as well differentiated (≥90%) or poorly differentiated (≤10%), depending on the degree to which neoplastic cells resemble their nonneoplastic counterparts. Grade is determined by measure of cellular proliferation using either Ki-67 immunolabeling indices or mitotic count (**Table 4**). Tumor grade and differentiation are closely related. In general, low-grade and intermediate-grade tumors are well differentiated, whereas high-grade tumors are poorly differentiated (see **Table 4**).[23,24] High-grade, poorly differentiated PNETs are very aggressive malignancies, with a biology and prognosis that parallel small cell carcinoma. These patients typically present with disseminated disease and should be managed with platinum-based chemotherapy. Rarely are patients with poorly differentiated PNETs surgical candidates.[25,26] On the other hand, well-differentiated PNETs follow a more indolent course, and treatment often involves a combination of surgical and nonsurgical therapies, as discussed later.

MANAGEMENT OF LOCOREGIONAL DISEASE

Surgical resection is the mainstay of therapy for patients who present with locoregional disease. Complete tumor extirpation offers the only opportunity for cure and provides symptomatic relief for patients with functional PNETs. With the exception of most insulinomas, most PNETs are malignant[7,8,27] and resection for these neoplasms should follow sound oncologic principles, including formal pancreatectomy and regional lymphadenectomy.[28,29] Depending on tumor location, pancreaticoduodenectomy, distal pancreatectomy, or total pancreatectomy is typically performed. For patients with benign insulinomas, laparoscopic or open enucleation is the procedure of choice.

Table 3					
Seventh edition AJCC staging and 5-year stage-specific survival for PNETs					

Primary Tumor

Tx: primary tumor cannot be assessed
T0: no evidence of primary tumor
Tis: carcinoma in situ
T1: tumor limited to pancreas, ≤2 cm in greatest dimension
T2: tumor limited to pancreas, >2 cm in greatest dimension
T3: tumor extends beyond pancreas but without celiac or SMA involvement
T4: tumor involves celiac axis or SMA (unresectable primary tumor)

Regional Lymph Nodes

NX: regional lymph nodes cannot be assessed
N0: no regional lymph node metastases
N1: regional lymph node metastases

Distant Metastases

M0: no distant metastases
M1: distant metastases

	Staging Classification			Stage-Specific 5-y Survival (%)	
Stage 0	Tis	N0	M0	Stage I	61
Stage IA	T1	N0	M0	Stage II	52
Stage IB	T2	N0	M0	Stage III	41
Stage IIA	T3	N0	M0	Stage IV	15
Stage IIB	T1-3	N1	M0		
Stage III	T4	Any N	M0		
Stage IV	Any T	Any N	M1		

Survival data are observed survival based on patients with PNET identified from the National Cancer Database in whom sixth edition AJCC criteria for pancreatic adenocarcinoma were applied.
Abbreviation: SMA, superior mesenteric artery.
From Bilimoria KY, Bentrem DJ, Merkow RP, et al. Application of the pancreatic adenocarcinoma staging system to pancreatic neuroendocrine tumors. J Am Coll Surg 2007;205(4):558–63.

Moreover, some groups have begun to explore the usefulness of enucleation plus regional lymphadenectomy for small (<2 cm), nonfunctional PNETs.[30,31]

Because of the lack of a hormonally mediated clinical syndrome, nonfunctional PNETs are often locally advanced at the time of diagnosis,[28,29,32] nevertheless, rates of resectability and survival are improved compared with pancreatic adenocarcinoma.[33] Institutional and population-based analyses have reported a median survival

Table 4			
Histopathologic classification of PNETs			
	Low Grade	**Intermediate Grade**	**High Grade**
Ki-67 index	<2%	2%–20%	>20%
Mitotic count	<2/50 HPF	2–20/50 HPF	>20/50 HPF
Differentiation	Well differentiated	Well differentiated	Poorly differentiated

Abbreviation: HPF, high power field.

of about 7 to 10 years for patients undergoing resection for locoregional disease.[32,34–36] However, data from the NCDB[21] and SEER[35] suggest that pancreatectomy, even for patients with localized disease, may be underused. Given the favorable overall survival and acceptable morbidity for pancreatectomy performed in experienced centers,[37] patients presenting with resectable tumors should be offered surgery for potential cure, provided they are otherwise appropriate operative candidates.

It is important to recognize the propensity for these tumors to metastasize after surgical extirpation of the primary lesion, with the liver being the most common site of recurrence. In a series reported from MD Anderson Cancer Center (MDACC) of 163 patients with nonfunctional PNETs, 42 underwent resection for localized disease. At a median follow-up of 2.7 years, 20 (48%) of these individuals had developed metachronous liver metastases.[32] Although PNETs are generally regarded as indolent tumors, recurrence after resection with curative intent is common; therefore, these patients require diligent oncologic surveillance. Current recommendations include postresection follow-up with physical examination, pertinent laboratory (tumor markers), and cross-sectional imaging at least biannually to annually.[38]

Patients who present with locally advanced, unresectable disease (ie, encasement of celiac or superior mesenteric arteries) in the absence of distant metastases require an individualized therapeutic strategy to provide optimal palliation. There are no data to support debulking or planned R2 resection of the primary tumor, and such an approach is likely to result in unnecessary morbidity. Occasionally, these patients may require palliative bypass operations to relieve biliary or gastric outlet obstruction. Furthermore, consideration should be given to select use of systemic as well as locoregional therapies to manage tumor progression or extrapancreatic metastases as they arise. In the MDACC series, this subset of patients had a median survival of 5.2 years.[32]

Management of Liver Metastases

Hepatic metastases occur in greater than 50% of patients with PNETs and are an important determinant of survival.[6,32,39,40] Historical controls indicate a 5-year survival of 30% to 40% if left untreated.[41,42] The armentarium of modalities available for the treatment of liver metastases continues to expand and outcomes are improved for those treated with an aggressive approach. The treatment of liver metastases may involve participation of surgeons, interventional radiologists, medical oncologists, and potentially nuclear medicine physicians. A management scheme for an individual patient should be based on the extent and distribution of liver lesions, symptom complex, status of the primary tumor, presence of extrahepatic metastases, and performance status.

HEPATIC RESECTION

If feasible, surgical resection of PNET liver metastases is preferred. Although complete resection is ideal and offers the only potential for cure, experience from the Mayo Clinic has shown that cytoreductive surgery, in which 90% or greater of tumor burden is cleared, provides benefit in both symptom control and survival.[43–45] In a report of 170 patients who underwent hepatectomy for neuroendocrine liver metastases, complete resection was achieved in 75 patients, whereas 95 patients had at least 90% cytoreduction.[44] Overall, 104 of 108 (96%) individuals with symptoms of hormone hypersecretion experienced relief; however, symptom recurrence rate was 59% at 5 years. Tumor recurrence rates were significantly prolonged in patients who underwent complete resection versus cytoreduction (76% vs 91% at 5 years). Five-year overall survival for the entire cohort was 61% (median survival 81 months). The Mayo data have been corroborated by other institutional series.[46–48] Although these studies are limited by inclusion of heterogeneous groups of patients as well as an element of selection bias, the collective experience shows that hepatectomy for neuroendocrine liver metastases effectively controls symptoms and improves survival. These findings, coupled with low morbidity and mortality associated with contemporary liver resection, support an aggressive surgical approach for patients with PNET liver metastases.

A more recent retrospective study from the Mayo Clinic reported their experience with hepatic resection exclusively in patients with sporadic, nonfunctional PNETs.[49] Among 72 patients identified, 54% underwent resection with curative intent and 44% with palliative intent (≥90% cytoreduction). Overall median survival for the entire study cohort was 7.4 years, with 1-year, 5-year, and 10-year survival rates of 97.1%, 59.9%, and 45%, respectively. Five-year overall survival was 69% in patients undergoing R0 resection versus 48% for those having 90% debulking or greater, although this figure did not reach statistical significance ($P = .07$). However, recurrence rates remain high even in patients undergoing R0 resection, with 1-year and 5-year disease-free survival of 53.7% and 10.7%, respectively.

For patients undergoing hepatic resection for metastatic PNET, careful preoperative planning is critical for optimizing outcomes. For example, in patients who present with synchronous liver metastases, cautious judgment is required when deciding whether to perform a combined procedure (simultaneous pancreatectomy and hepatectomy) versus a staged approach. Although performance of combined procedures is documented in the literature,[49,50] the potential morbidity of simultaneous pancreatectomy and major hepatectomy should be weighed carefully. In the Mayo Clinic series cited earlier, 51% morbidity was reported for patients undergoing simultaneous pancreatectomy and hepatectomy.[49] Given that these tumors often remain stable in size for several months, consideration should be given to performing staged resections for patients with synchronous liver metastases, particularly if a major hepatic resection (≥4 segments) is required.

LOCAL ABLATIVE TECHNIQUES

Local ablative techniques have a role in the treatment of PNET liver metastases that are surgically inaccessible. Although several forms of therapy such as cryoablation and percutaneous ethanol injection have been reported,[51] radiofrequency ablation (RFA) is the preferred technique in most centers.[51–53] It can be performed during open or laparoscopic surgery (alone or in conjunction with resection) or via a percutaneous approach. In a 10-year experience of laparoscopic RFA for neuroendocrine liver metastases (including 18 patients with PNET), the Cleveland Clinic reported significant or complete symptom relief in 70% of patients, median duration of symptom control of 11 months, and 5-year survival of 48% after application of RFA.[54] In addition to RFA, microwave ablation is increasingly used for ablation of primary and secondary liver tumors and has been shown to have a role in the management of neuroendocrine liver metastases.[55] Although surgical resection, if technically feasible, is the treatment of choice for PNET liver metastases, local ablation serves as an effective adjunct or alternative therapy in the treatment of these patients.[48,49]

HEPATIC ARTERIAL EMBOLIZATION PROCEDURES

Patients with diffuse, unresectable liver metastases may be candidates for hepatic arterial embolization procedures.[56] The rationale for these techniques is that hepatic metastases derive their blood supply from hepatic arterial circulation, whereas normal liver parenchyma is supplied primarily by portal venous flow. After selective arterial catheterization, embolization can be performed with a variety of occlusive particles introduced either alone (bland embolization) or after infusion of a suspension containing a cytotoxic agent (chemoembolization), such as doxorubicin, streptozosin, or cisplatin. There are no randomized studies comparing bland embolization versus chemoembolization. Reported response rates, derived primarily from retrospective institutional series,[57–59] indicate that these techniques are relatively equivalent. In a review of patients treated at MDACC, Gupta and colleagues[60] analyzed outcomes based on both location of the primary tumor and type of embolization performed. In this series, univariate analysis revealed a trend toward improved survival and response rate in PNET patients treated with chemoembolization versus bland embolization. These data do not definitively support the use of chemoembolization over bland embolization for PNET metastases. However, given the sensitivity of PNETs to systemic chemotherapy (as opposed to relatively chemoresistant midgut carcinoids), it seems reasonable that chemoembolization may be preferred over bland embolization in patients with PNET liver metastases. Contraindications for performing hepatic arterial embolization include portal vein thrombosis and hepatic insufficiency.[56]

A more recently developed form of liver-directed therapy available for patients with neuroendocrine liver metastases is Y^{90} (a β-emitting particle) radioembolization.[61] This technique uses radioactive yttrium embedded either in resin or glass microspheres, which are delivered via selective arterial catheterization. Unlike hepatic arterial embolization and chemoembolization, complete arterial occlusion and tumor ischemia are not the goal, because radiotherapy has its optimal effects under normal oxygen tension. The efficacy of this approach has been reported in several recent studies.[62–64] In a collaborative, retrospective analysis of 148 patients from several centers in the United States and Europe, radiographic response rates were about 60% and minimal toxicity was reported.[62] As opposed to bland or chemoembolization procedures, which often require a 2-day to 3-day hospital admission, radioembolization is typically performed in the outpatient setting, and repeat procedures may be performed in some circumstances.[61]

LIVER TRANSPLANTATION

In the setting of diffuse, unresectable neuroendocrine liver metastases refractory to other lines of therapy, orthotopic liver transplantation (OLT) may be considered for select patients. OLT may permit excellent symptom relief in patients with life-threatening hormonal disturbances and potentially offer cure in patients with metastases confined to the liver.[65] Disease recurrence is common and long-term survival less than optimal. In a meta-analysis of 103 patients having transplantation for neuroendocrine liver metastases, 5-year overall and disease-free survival were 47% and 24%, respectively.[66] Although several subsequent institutional series have reported higher 5-year overall survival,[67–69] cure is exceedingly rare. Criteria proposed to better select OLT candidates and optimize outcomes include age younger than 50 years,[66] low grade (as determined by Ki-67 index), tumors that stain for epithelial cadherin,[69] and metastatic diffusion to 50% or less of hepatic parenchyma.[70] Given limited donor resources, and low cure rates observed in reported series, OLT for patients with metastatic PNET should undergo continued investigation with efforts aimed at refining selection criteria.

MEDICAL THERAPIES FOR ADVANCED DISEASE
Cytotoxic Chemotherapy

Current systemic therapies for patients with locally advanced, unresectable or metastatic PNETs include both cytotoxic chemotherapy and molecular targeted agents.

Historically, streptozotocin-based regimens have been the standard chemotherapy for patients with advanced disease. Initial trials by Moertel and colleagues[71,72] reported response rates greater than 60% using combination therapies of streptozotocin with either 5-fluorouracil (5-FU) or doxorubicin. However, criteria used to evaluate response in these early studies were not well standardized, and subsequent reports have failed to show such robust efficacy.[73–75] In a review of 84 patients treated with combination of streptozotocin, 5-FU, and doxorubicin, Kouvaraki and colleagues[74] documented a response of 39% (using RECIST [Response Evaluation Criteria in Solid Tumors]), and a 2-year progression-free and overall survival of 41% and 74%, respectively.

More recent studies have evaluated efficacy of the oral alkylating agent temozolomide in patients with advanced PNETs. When used in combination with targeted therapies, objective response rates of 24% to 45% have been observed.[76–78] Moreover, a recent retrospective analysis of 30 patients treated with combination capecitabine (oral prodrug of 5-FU) and temozolomide documented an objective response rate of 70%, with minimal toxicity when compared with traditional streptozosin-based regimens.[79] The marked response observed in this study is believed to result, in part, from capecitabine-induced depletion of DNA repair enzymes, resulting in increased sensitivity of tumor cells to temozolomide. Although streptozosin remains the only cytotoxic agent approved by the US Food and Drug Administration (FDA) for patients with advanced PNET, the efficacy of temozolomide reported in these studies warrants its consideration for use in clinical protocols and potential phase III trials.

Molecular Targeted Therapies

Recent progress in the treatment of patients with neuroendocrine tumors has come through the application of molecular targeted therapies. In particular, inhibitors of the mammalian target of rapamycin (mTOR) and multireceptor targeted tyrosine kinase inhibitors (TKIs) have shown improvements in progression-free survival when used in patients with advanced PNETs.[80]

The intracellular serine-threonine kinase mTOR plays a key role in cell growth and proliferation, cellular metabolism, and apoptosis. Although there are no documented mTOR mutations, there are several lines of evidence that the upregulation of mTOR activity plays a role in the development and growth of neuroendocrine tumors.[81] Studies evaluating the efficacy of mTOR inhibitors in patients with advanced disease have shown encouraging results.[82–84] A recent large, randomized, placebo-controlled trial in patients with advanced PNETs reported significant improvement in progression-free survival (11 months vs 4.6 months, $P<.001$) in patients treated with the mTOR inhibitor everolimus.[84] Based on results of this trial, everolimus became the first agent in more than 30 years to receive FDA approval for the treatment of locally advanced, unresectable or metastatic PNET.

PNETs are highly vascular tumors and dependence on vascular endothelial growth factor (VEGF) is known to play a critical role in their development and progression.[85] Small-molecule TKIs such as pazopanib, sorafenib, and sunitinib, which block VEGF activity, have been studied in patients with advanced neuroendocrine tumors.[86–88] A recent multicenter, double-blind, placebo-controlled trial examined the role of sunitinib in patients with locally advanced, unresectable or metastatic PNET.[89] Although this trial was discontinued before planned interim analysis, among evaluable patients there was a significant improvement in progression-free survival (11.4 months vs 5.5 months, $P<.001$) and objective tumor response (9.3% vs 0%, $P = .007$) for patients in the sunitinib arm. Based on these data, sunitinib also recently received FDA approval as a first-line therapy for patients with advanced PNET. In addition to TKIs, the anti-VEGF monoclonal antibody, bevacizumab, also seems to have usefulness in the treatment of patients with advanced neuroendocrine tumors when used in combination with other targeted agents[90] or cytotoxic chemotherapy.[91]

Somatostatin Analogues and Peptide Receptor Radiotherapy

As mentioned earlier, most neuroendocrine tumors overexpress somatostatin receptors. Somatostatin analogues such as octreotide and lanreotide are effective at ameliorating symptoms in patients with functional tumors. Although robust tumor regression is not expected, these agents do seem to have a cytostatic effect that may result in disease stabilization, even in the metastatic setting.[92–94] The recent placebo controlled, double blind, prospective, randomized study on the effect of octreotide LAR in the control of tumor growth in patients with metastatic neuroendocrine midgut tumors (PROMID Study) reported that long-acting octreotide results in significant progression-free survival in patients with midgut carcinoids.[94] Whether these agents have similar antiproliferative properties in advanced PNETs has not been determined in a prospective fashion.

Peptide receptor radiotherapy (PRRT) is an emerging technique for patients with metastatic, unresectable, somatostatin receptor positive tumors.[95,96] A radioisotope such as yttrium-90 or luteticium-177 is coupled with a somatostatin analogue that is administered systemically and permits selective delivery of cytotoxic doses of radioactivity to tumor cells. In a Dutch study of 504 patients receiving PRRT for advanced neuroendocrine tumors, 310 were evaluated for efficacy. Objective radiographic response was observed in 46% of patients and disease stabilization in 35%.[97] Response rates in patients with gastrinomas, insulinomas, VIPomas and nonfunctioning PNETs were higher than in patients with carcinoid tumors. Multivariate analysis reported high-intensity uptake on octreoscan and a Karnofsky performance status 70 or greater as positive predictors of response to therapy. Grade 3 or 4 toxicity was observed in 11.3% of patients and included acute hematologic toxicities or delayed toxicity in the form of renal insufficiency, liver failure, or myelodysplastic syndrome. Given the encouraging response rates observed and acceptable toxicity profile, PRRT seems to be a promising tool in the management of patients with advanced neuroendocrine tumors. Although approved for use in Europe, this form of therapy remains investigational in the United States.

Future Directions

Although the hereditary neuroendocrine syndromes are rare, advances made in understanding their genetic alterations has begun to shed some light on the molecular pathogenesis of the more common sporadic tumors.

For instance, 25% to 30% of sporadic PNETs harbor a somatic inactivating mutation of the *MEN1* gene on 1 allele combined with loss of the second allele.[23,98] In addition, mutations in *TSC2* (involved in the development of tuberous sclerosis complex) result in upregulation of mTOR activity and seem to lead to a more aggressive tumor phenotype as shown by higher proliferation indices, increased liver metastases, and decreased progression-free survival.[81] In a recent study by Jiao and colleagues,[1] exomic sequencing in 68 sporadic PNETs revealed mutations of *MEN1*, *DAXX/ATRX*, and genes involved in the mTOR pathway in 44%, 43%, and 14%, respectively. Patients with mutations in the *MEN1* and *DAXX/ATRX* genes had a significantly improved survival compared with patients with wild-type alleles at these sites. This type of data will help better understand the natural history of this disease and prognosis for certain subsets of patients. Furthermore, identifying patients with mutations in the mTOR pathway may provide improved selection of patients to receive treatment with mTOR inhibitors. Because of the rarity of these neoplasms and paucity of well-controlled trials comparing the efficacy of various treatment modalities, the management of patients with advanced disease remains largely empirical. Moreover, appropriate management of small (≤2 cm), asymptomatic, incidentally found PNETs remains unclear. Should these patients have radical resection, laparoscopic enucleation, or is observation with serial imaging safe? As further characterization of the molecular underpinnings of PNETs continues, it is likely to translate into improved clinical decision making in these areas of uncertainty.

SUMMARY

PNETs account for 1% to 2% of pancreatic neoplasms and may occur sporadically or as part of a hereditary syndrome. Patients may present with symptoms related to hormone secretion by functional tumors or from symptoms related to locally advanced or metastatic nonfunctional tumors. Moreover, asymptomatic PNETs are increasingly detected incidentally during abdominal imaging performed for other reasons. The management of localized PNETs is surgical resection. However, most patients experience distant metastases and require a well-coordinated multidisciplinary effort to optimize outcomes. Hepatic metastases are common and their management involves a variety of liver-directed therapies, which should be tailored according to extent of disease, symptoms, presence of extrahepatic metastases, and patient performance status. Systemic therapy for patients with advanced disease has historically been limited to streptozosin-based regimens; however, newer cytotoxic agents such as temozolomide seem to have equal, if not improved, antitumor efficacy. In addition, progress in the application of molecular targeted therapies has led to recent FDA approval of the mTOR inhibitor, everolimus, and the multitargeted TKI sunitinib for patients with advanced disease. Therapies such as PRRT have shown promise in the treatment of patients with metastatic disease and will likely undergo formal investigation in the United States in the near future. In parallel with the development of new treatment strategies, significant work is taking place to better understand the molecular pathogenesis of PNETs, which will contribute to a better understanding of their natural history and, it is hoped, begin to guide the selection of therapy for particular patients. Heterogeneity in the presentation and biological behavior of PNETs can present unique clinical challenges; therefore, it is important for clinicians involved in their management to be aware of the various treatment options and work in concert to develop an optimal therapeutic strategy for the individual patient.

REFERENCES

1. Jiao Y, Shi C, Edil BH, et al. DAXX/ATRX, MEN1, and mTOR pathway genes are frequently altered in pancreatic neuroendocrine tumors. Science 2011; 331(6021):1199–203.
2. Vosburgh E. Tumors of the diffuse neuroendocrine and gastroenteropancreatic endocrine system. In: Hong W, Bast RC, editors. Cancer medicine. 8th edition. Shelton (CT): People's Medical Publishing House-USA; 2010. p. 940–58.
3. Exocrine and endocrine pancreas. In: Edge S, Byrd DR, editors. AJCC cancer staging manual. 7th edition. New York: Springer; 2010. p. 241–9.
4. Rindi G, Bordi C. Endocrine tumours of the gastrointestinal tract: aetiology, molecular pathogenesis and genetics. Best Pract Res Clin Gastroenterol 2005;19(4): 519–34.
5. Rindi G, Wiedenmann B. Neuroendocrine neoplasms of the gut and pancreas: new insights. Nat Rev Endocrinol 2011;8(1):54–64.

6. Yao JC, Eisner MP, Leary C, et al. Population-based study of islet cell carcinoma. Ann Surg Oncol 2007;14(12):3492–500.
7. Metz DC, Jensen RT. Gastrointestinal neuroendocrine tumors: pancreatic endocrine tumors. Gastroenterology 2008;135(5):1469–92.
8. Kulke MH, Anthony LB, Bushnell DL, et al. NANETS treatment guidelines: well-differentiated neuroendocrine tumors of the stomach and pancreas. Pancreas 2010;39(6):735–52.
9. Oberg K, Eriksson B. Endocrine tumours of the pancreas. Best Pract Res Clin Gastroenterol 2005;19(5):753–81.
10. Plockinger U, Wiedenmann B. Diagnosis of non-functioning neuro-endocrine gastro-enteropancreatic tumours. Neuroendocrinology 2004;80(Suppl 1):35–8.
11. Campana D, Nori F, Piscitelli L, et al. Chromogranin A: is it a useful marker of neuroendocrine tumors? J Clin Oncol 2007;25(15):1967–73.
12. Seregni E, Ferrari L, Bajetta E, et al. Clinical significance of blood chromogranin A measurement in neuroendocrine tumours. Ann Oncol 2001;12(Suppl 2): S69–72.
13. Stivanello M, Berruti A, Torta M, et al. Circulating chromogranin A in the assessment of patients with neuroendocrine tumours. A single institution experience. Ann Oncol 2001;12(Suppl 2):S73–7.
14. Jensen RT, Berna MJ, Bingham DB, et al. Inherited pancreatic endocrine tumor syndromes: advances in molecular pathogenesis, diagnosis, management, and controversies. Cancer 2008;113(Suppl 7):1807–43.
15. Rockall AG, Reznek RH. Imaging of neuroendocrine tumours (CT/MR/US). Best Pract Res Clin Endocrinol Metab 2007;21(1):43–68.
16. Anderson MA, Carpenter S, Thompson NW, et al. Endoscopic ultrasound is highly accurate and directs management in patients with neuroendocrine tumors of the pancreas. Am J Gastroenterol 2000;95(9):2271–7.
17. Sundin A, Garske U, Orlefors H. Nuclear imaging of neuroendocrine tumours. Best Pract Res Clin Endocrinol Metab 2007;21(1):69–85.
18. Virgolini I, Traub-Weidinger T, Decristoforo C. Nuclear medicine in the detection and management of pancreatic islet-cell tumours. Best Pract Res Clin Endocrinol Metab 2005;19(2):213–27.
19. Kloppel G, Perren A, Heitz PU. The gastroenteropancreatic neuroendocrine cell system and its tumors: the WHO classification. Ann N Y Acad Sci 2004;1014:13–27.
20. Rindi G, Kloppel G, Alhman H, et al. TNM staging of foregut (neuro)endocrine tumors: a consensus proposal including a grading system. Virchows Arch 2006;449(4):395–401.
21. Bilimoria KY, Bentrem DJ, Merkow RP, et al. Application of the pancreatic adenocarcinoma staging system to pancreatic neuroendocrine tumors. J Am Coll Surg 2007;205(4):558–63.
22. Halfdanarson TR, Rabe KG, Rubin J, et al. Pancreatic neuroendocrine tumors (PNETs): incidence, prognosis and recent trend toward improved survival. Ann Oncol 2008;19(10):1727–33.
23. Capelli P, Martignoni G, Pedica F, et al. Endocrine neoplasms of the pancreas: pathologic and genetic features. Arch Pathol Lab Med 2009;133(3):350–64.
24. Pape UF, Jann H, Muller-Nordhorn J, et al. Prognostic relevance of a novel TNM classification system for upper gastroenteropancreatic neuroendocrine tumors. Cancer 2008;113(2):256–65.
25. Klimstra DS, Modlin IR, Coppola D, et al. The pathologic classification of neuroendocrine tumors: a review of nomenclature, grading, and staging systems. Pancreas 2010;39(6):707–12.

26. Strosberg JR, Coppola D, Klimstra DS, et al. The NANETS consensus guidelines for the diagnosis and management of poorly differentiated (high-grade) extrapulmonary neuroendocrine carcinomas. Pancreas 2010;39(6):799–800.
27. Falconi M, Plockinger U, Kwekkeboom DJ, et al. Well-differentiated pancreatic nonfunctioning tumors/carcinoma. Neuroendocrinology 2006;84(3):196–211.
28. Fendrich V, Bartsch DK. Surgical treatment of gastrointestinal neuroendocrine tumors. Langenbecks Arch Surg 2011;396(3):299–311.
29. Kouvaraki MA, Solorzano CC, Shapiro SE, et al. Surgical treatment of non-functioning pancreatic islet cell tumors. J Surg Oncol 2005;89(3):170–85.
30. Fernandez-Cruz L, Molina V, Vallejos R, et al. Outcome after laparoscopic enucleation for non-functional neuroendocrine pancreatic tumours. HPB (Oxford) 2012; 14(3):171–6.
31. Zerbi A, Capitanio V, Boninsegna L, et al. Surgical treatment of pancreatic endocrine tumours in Italy: results of a prospective multicentre study of 262 cases. Langenbecks Arch Surg 2011;396(3):313–21.
32. Solorzano CC, Lee JE, Pisters PW, et al. Nonfunctioning islet cell carcinoma of the pancreas: survival results in a contemporary series of 163 patients. Surgery 2001; 130(6):1078–85.
33. Hodul PJ, Strosberg JR, Kvols LK. Aggressive surgical resection in the management of pancreatic neuroendocrine tumors: when is it indicated? Cancer Control 2008;15(4):314–21.
34. Grant CS. Surgical management of malignant islet cell tumors. World J Surg 1993;17(4):498–503.
35. Hill JS, McPhee JT, McDade TP, et al. Pancreatic neuroendocrine tumors: the impact of surgical resection on survival. Cancer 2009;115(4):741–51.
36. Schurr PG, Strate T, Rese K, et al. Aggressive surgery improves long-term survival in neuroendocrine pancreatic tumors: an institutional experience. Ann Surg 2007;245(2):273–81.
37. Birkmeyer JD, Siewers AE, Finlayson EV, et al. Hospital volume and surgical mortality in the United States. N Engl J Med 2002;346(15):1128–37.
38. Kulke MH, Benson AB 3rd, Bergsland E, et al. Neuroendocrine tumors. J Natl Compr Canc Netw 2012;10(6):724–64.
39. Ekeblad S, Skogseid B, Dunder K, et al. Prognostic factors and survival in 324 patients with pancreatic endocrine tumor treated at a single institution. Clin Cancer Res 2008;14(23):7798–803.
40. Tomassetti P, Campana D, Piscitelli L, et al. Endocrine pancreatic tumors: factors correlated with survival. Ann Oncol 2005;16(11):1806–10.
41. Moertel CG. Karnofsky memorial lecture. An odyssey in the land of small tumors. J Clin Oncol 1987;5(10):1502–22.
42. Thompson GB, van Heerden JA, Grant CS, et al. Islet cell carcinomas of the pancreas: a twenty-year experience. Surgery 1988;104(6):1011–7.
43. Que FG, Nagorney DM, Batts KP, et al. Hepatic resection for metastatic neuroendocrine carcinomas. Am J Surg 1995;169(1):36–42 [discussion: 42–3].
44. Sarmiento JM, Heywood G, Rubin J, et al. Surgical treatment of neuroendocrine metastases to the liver: a plea for resection to increase survival. J Am Coll Surg 2003;197(1):29–37.
45. Sarmiento JM, Que FG. Hepatic surgery for metastases from neuroendocrine tumors. Surg Oncol Clin N Am 2003;12(1):231–42.
46. Chamberlain RS, Canes D, Brown KT, et al. Hepatic neuroendocrine metastases: does intervention alter outcomes? J Am Coll Surg 2000;190(4):432–45.

47. Elias D, Lasser P, Ducreux M, et al. Liver resection (and associated extrahepatic resections) for metastatic well-differentiated endocrine tumors: a 15-year single center prospective study. Surgery 2003;133(4):375–82.

48. Glazer ES, Tseng JF, Al-Refaie W, et al. Long-term survival after surgical management of neuroendocrine hepatic metastases. HPB (Oxford) 2010;12(6):427–33.

49. Cusati D, Zhang L, Harmsen WS, et al. Metastatic nonfunctioning pancreatic neuroendocrine carcinoma to liver: surgical treatment and outcomes. J Am Coll Surg 2012;215(1):117–24.

50. Gaujoux S, Gonen M, Tang L, et al. Synchronous resection of primary and liver metastases for neuroendocrine tumors. Ann Surg Oncol 2012;19(13):4270–7.

51. Sheen AJ, Poston GJ, Sherlock DJ. Cryotherapeutic ablation of liver tumours. Br J Surg 2002;89(11):1396–401.

52. Siperstein AE, Berber E. Cryoablation, percutaneous alcohol injection, and radiofrequency ablation for treatment of neuroendocrine liver metastases. World J Surg 2001;25(6):693–6.

53. Steinmuller T, Kianmanesh R, Falconi M, et al. Consensus guidelines for the management of patients with liver metastases from digestive (neuro)endocrine tumors: foregut, midgut, hindgut, and unknown primary. Neuroendocrinology 2008;87(1): 47–62.

54. Mazzaglia PJ, Berber E, Milas M, et al. Laparoscopic radiofrequency ablation of neuroendocrine liver metastases: a 10-year experience evaluating predictors of survival. Surgery 2007;142(1):10–9.

55. Martin RC, Scoggins CR, McMasters KM. Safety and efficacy of microwave ablation of hepatic tumors: a prospective review of a 5-year experience. Ann Surg Oncol 2010;17(1):171–8.

56. Ruszniewski P, Malka D. Hepatic arterial chemoembolization in the management of advanced digestive endocrine tumors. Digestion 2000;62(Suppl 1):79–83.

57. Eriksson BK, Larsson EG, Skogseid BM, et al. Liver embolizations of patients with malignant neuroendocrine gastrointestinal tumors. Cancer 1998;83(11):2293–301.

58. Ruszniewski P, Rougier P, Roche A, et al. Hepatic arterial chemoembolization in patients with liver metastases of endocrine tumors. A prospective phase II study in 24 patients. Cancer 1993;71(8):2624–30.

59. Strosberg JR, Choi J, Cantor AB, et al. Selective hepatic artery embolization for treatment of patients with metastatic carcinoid and pancreatic endocrine tumors. Cancer Control 2006;13(1):72–8.

60. Gupta S, Johnson MM, Murthy R, et al. Hepatic arterial embolization and chemoembolization for the treatment of patients with metastatic neuroendocrine tumors: variables affecting response rates and survival. Cancer 2005;104(8):1590–602.

61. Vyleta M, Coldwell D. Radioembolization in the treatment of neuroendocrine tumor metastases to the liver. Int J Hepatol 2011;2011:785315.

62. Kennedy AS, Dezarn WA, McNeillie P, et al. Radioembolization for unresectable neuroendocrine hepatic metastases using resin 90Y-microspheres: early results in 148 patients. Am J Clin Oncol 2008;31(3):271–9.

63. King J, Quinn R, Glenn DM, et al. Radioembolization with selective internal radiation microspheres for neuroendocrine liver metastases. Cancer 2008;113(5):921–9.

64. Rhee TK, Lewandowski RJ, Liu DM, et al. 90Y Radioembolization for metastatic neuroendocrine liver tumors: preliminary results from a multi-institutional experience. Ann Surg 2008;247(6):1029–35.

65. Chan G, Kocha W, Reid R, et al. Liver transplantation for symptomatic liver metastases of neuroendocrine tumours. Curr Oncol 2012;19(4):217–21.

66. Lehnert T. Liver transplantation for metastatic neuroendocrine carcinoma: an analysis of 103 patients. Transplantation 1998;66(10):1307–12.
67. Frilling A, Malago M, Weber F, et al. Liver transplantation for patients with metastatic endocrine tumors: single-center experience with 15 patients. Liver Transpl 2006;12(7):1089–96.
68. Olausson M, Friman S, Herlenius G, et al. Orthotopic liver or multivisceral transplantation as treatment of metastatic neuroendocrine tumors. Liver Transpl 2007; 13(3):327–33.
69. Rosenau J, Bahr MJ, von Wasielewski R, et al. Ki67, E-cadherin, and p53 as prognostic indicators of long-term outcome after liver transplantation for metastatic neuroendocrine tumors. Transplantation 2002;73(3):386–94.
70. Mazzaferro V, Pulvirenti A, Coppa J. Neuroendocrine tumors metastatic to the liver: how to select patients for liver transplantation? J Hepatol 2007;47(4):460–6.
71. Moertel CG, Hanley JA, Johnson LA. Streptozocin alone compared with streptozocin plus fluorouracil in the treatment of advanced islet-cell carcinoma. N Engl J Med 1980;303(21):1189–94.
72. Moertel CG, Lefkopoulo M, Lipsitz S, et al. Streptozocin-doxorubicin, streptozocin-fluorouracil or chlorozotocin in the treatment of advanced islet-cell carcinoma. N Engl J Med 1992;326(8):519–23.
73. Cheng PN, Saltz LB. Failure to confirm major objective antitumor activity for streptozocin and doxorubicin in the treatment of patients with advanced islet cell carcinoma. Cancer 1999;86(6):944–8.
74. Kouvaraki MA, Ajani JA, Hoff P, et al. Fluorouracil, doxorubicin, and streptozocin in the treatment of patients with locally advanced and metastatic pancreatic endocrine carcinomas. J Clin Oncol 2004;22(23):4762–71.
75. McCollum AD, Kulke MH, Ryan DP, et al. Lack of efficacy of streptozocin and doxorubicin in patients with advanced pancreatic endocrine tumors. Am J Clin Oncol 2004;27(5):485–8.
76. Kulke MH, Stuart K, Enzinger PC, et al. Phase II study of temozolomide and thalidomide in patients with metastatic neuroendocrine tumors. J Clin Oncol 2006;24(3):401–6.
77. Kulke MH, Blaszkowsky L, Zhu A. Phase I/II study of everolimus (RAD001) in combination with temozolomide in patients with advanced pancreatic neuroendocrine tumors [abstract]. Gastroinestinal Cancers Symposium 2010;223a.
78. Chan JA, Stuart K, Earle CC, et al. Prospective study of bevacizumab plus temozolamide in patients with advanced neuroendocrine tumors. J Clin Oncol 2012; 30(24):2963–8.
79. Strosberg JR, Fine RL, Choi J, et al. First-line chemotherapy with capecitabine and temozolomide in patients with metastatic pancreatic endocrine carcinomas. Cancer 2011;117(2):268–75.
80. Jensen RT, Delle Fave G. Promising advances in the treatment of malignant pancreatic endocrine tumors. N Engl J Med 2011;364(6):564–5.
81. Missiaglia E, Dalai I, Barbi S, et al. Pancreatic endocrine tumors: expression profiling evidences a role for AKT-mTOR pathway. J Clin Oncol 2010;28(2): 245–55.
82. Duran I, Kortmansky J, Singh D, et al. A phase II clinical and pharmacodynamic study of temsirolimus in advanced neuroendocrine carcinomas. Br J Cancer 2006;95(9):1148–54.
83. Yao JC, Phan AT, Chang DZ, et al. Efficacy of RAD001 (everolimus) and octreotide LAR in advanced low- to intermediate-grade neuroendocrine tumors: results of a phase II study. J Clin Oncol 2008;26(26):4311–8.

84. Yao JC, Shah MH, Ito T, et al. Everolimus for advanced pancreatic neuroendocrine tumors. N Engl J Med 2011;364(6):514–23.
85. Zhang J, Jia Z, Li Q, et al. Elevated expression of vascular endothelial growth factor correlates with increased angiogenesis and decreased progression-free survival among patients with low-grade neuroendocrine tumors. Cancer 2007; 109(8):1478–86.
86. Hobday TR, Rubin J, Holen K, et al. MC044h, a phase II trial of sorafenib in patients with metastatic neuroendocrine tumors: a phase II consortium study [abstract]. ASCO Annual Meeting Proc 2007;25:4505a.
87. Kulke MH, Lenz HJ, Meropol NJ, et al. Activity of sunitinib in patients with advanced neuroendocrine tumors. J Clin Oncol 2008;26(20):3403–10.
88. Phan A, Yao J, Fogelman D. A prospective, multi-institutional phase II study of GW786034 (pazopanib) and depot octreotide in advanced low-grade neuroendocrine carcinoma [abstract]. J Clin Oncol 2010;28:15s.
89. Raymond E, Dahan L, Raoul JL, et al. Sunitinib malate for the treatment of pancreatic neuroendocrine tumors. N Engl J Med 2011;364(6):501–13.
90. Yao JC, Phan A, Fogelman D, et al. Randomized run-in study of bevacizumab (B) and everolimus (E) in low- to intermediate-grade neuroendocrine tumors (LGNETs) using perfusion CT as functional biomarker. J Clin Oncol 2010; 28(Suppl 15):4002.
91. Kunz PL, Kou T, Zahn JM, et al. A phase II study of capecitabine, oxaliplatin, and bevacizumab for metastatic or unresectable neuroendocrine tumors. J Clin Oncol 2010;28(Suppl 15):4104.
92. Butturini G, Bettini R, Missiaglia E, et al. Predictive factors of efficacy of the somatostatin analogue octreotide as first line therapy for advanced pancreatic endocrine carcinoma. Endocr Relat Cancer 2006;13(4):1213–21.
93. Panzuto F, Di Fonzo M, Iannicelli E, et al. Long-term clinical outcome of somatostatin analogues for treatment of progressive, metastatic, well-differentiated entero-pancreatic endocrine carcinoma. Ann Oncol 2006;17(3):461–6.
94. Rinke A, Muller HH, Schade-Brittinger C, et al. Placebo-controlled, double-blind, prospective, randomized study on the effect of octreotide LAR in the control of tumor growth in patients with metastatic neuroendocrine midgut tumors: a report from the PROMID Study Group. J Clin Oncol 2009;27(28):4656–63.
95. Kwekkeboom DJ, de Herder WW, Krenning EP. Somatostatin receptor-targeted radionuclide therapy in patients with gastroenteropancreatic neuroendocrine tumors. Endocrinol Metab Clin North Am 2011;40(1):173–85, ix.
96. Nicolas G, Giovacchini G, Muller-Brand J, et al. Targeted radiotherapy with radiolabeled somatostatin analogs. Endocrinol Metab Clin North Am 2011;40(1): 187–204, ix–x.
97. Kwekkeboom DJ, de Herder WW, Kam BL, et al. Treatment with the radiolabeled somatostatin analog [177 Lu-DOTA 0, Tyr3]octreotate: toxicity, efficacy, and survival. J Clin Oncol 2008;26(13):2124–30.
98. Corbo V, Dalai I, Scardoni M, et al. MEN1 in pancreatic endocrine tumors: analysis of gene and protein status in 169 sporadic neoplasms reveals alterations in the vast majority of cases. Endocr Relat Cancer 2010;17(3):771–83.

Quality Metrics in Pancreatic Surgery

Somala Mohammed, MD[a,b], William E. Fisher, MD[b,*]

KEYWORDS

• Pancreatectomy • Outcomes • Pancreaticoduodenectomy • Quality metrics

KEY POINTS

• The quality of pancreatic surgery is variable. Outcomes are superior when pancreatico-duodenectomy is performed by high-volume pancreatic surgeons practicing in hospitals with a high volume of pancreatic surgery.

• Training qualified pancreatic surgeons takes time. A long learning curve exists in pancreatic surgery and measurable outcomes are improved by frequent repetition.

• Mortality following pancreaticoduodenectomy has improved in recent decades and currently should be an uncommon event (<5%).

• Pancreas surgeons and the institutions where they practice should track and report quality metrics. Collection of quality metrics requires organization, attention to detail, and investment.

• National benchmarking data will soon be available to assist pancreatic surgeons and hospitals in assessing the quality of pancreatic surgery.

INTRODUCTION

Outcomes after pancreatic surgery have improved over the decades, but morbidity remains high. Pancreatic surgery is complex and, as it continues to evolve, the measurement of short-term and long-term outcomes becomes increasingly important. However, acquiring accurate surgeon-specific or hospital-specific data for systematic comparison of outcomes remains a challenge, and the data on performance that do exist are variable. Furthermore, few established quality metrics in this field currently exist. Many institutional experiences have been published over the years. Although these reviews provide a general idea of the state of pancreatic surgery and share a set of potential benchmarks against which other pancreatic surgeons can assess

There are no disclosures for either author.
[a] Division of General Surgery, Michael E. DeBakey Department of Surgery, Baylor College of Medicine, One Baylor Plaza, Suite 404D, Houston, TX 77030, USA; [b] Elkins Pancreas Cente, Baylor College of Medicine, 6620 Main Street, Suite 1450, Houston, TX 77030, USA
* Corresponding author.
E-mail address: wfisher@bcm.edu

themselves, they collectively show wide variability in short-term outcomes, long-term survival, quality of life, and use of quality metrics.[1]

Over the past several decades, the safety and demand for pancreatic surgery have increased. For example, an increasing number of pancreaticoduodenectomies are being performed for indications other than pancreatic ductal adenocarcinoma, such as premalignant pancreatic cysts or cystic neoplasms, pancreatitis or its complications, endocrine tumors, and cancers of the surrounding biliary ductal system or gastrointestinal tract. Some centers also offer resection to patients with tumors of borderline resectability after neoadjuvant therapy, and the possibility of venous reconstruction has provided surgical opportunities for patients who previously would not have undergone resection.

With the advent of minimally invasive and robot-assisted surgical technology, there is potential for further advances in the field. Although not as rapidly or widely adopted as laparoscopic approaches for most other general surgical procedures, outcomes with these technologically advanced surgeries are being explored by some pancreatic surgeons. Data on laparoscopic distal pancreatectomies for patients with benign lesions seems to validate the approach as acceptable and safe with the added inherent benefits of the laparoscopic technique, such as potentially lower intraoperative blood loss, less postoperative pain and analgesic requirements, earlier return of bowel function, and shorter recovery and hospital stay.[2] Robot-assisted laparoscopic pancreaticoduodenectomy is starting to be offered to patients at specialized pancreas centers throughout the world as well. However, these promising minimally invasive procedures require further systematic evaluation with defined quality metrics so that outcomes can be compared with traditional, open approaches before widespread adoption.

As indications for pancreatic surgery expand, and increasingly complex technologies are used, pancreatic surgeons are seeking metrics to monitor outcomes and assess quality. Surgeons have always been interested in comparing their outcomes with those of others, but the need for valid quality metrics is intensifying. With the health care system's growing emphasis on paying for performance, systematic assessment of quality and outcomes, including cost, in surgery is imperative. Such endeavors will allow greater insight into common challenges that face practitioners and ultimately contribute to further improvements in patient care.

THE IMPACT OF VOLUME ON POSTOPERATIVE OUTCOMES

A relationship between operative volume and improved outcomes in pancreatic surgery has been shown in numerous studies. Lieberman and colleagues[3] investigated the effect of hospital and surgeon volume on perioperative deaths after pancreaticoduodenectomy or total pancreatectomy performed in New York State from 1984 to 1991 for peripancreatic cancer. This group showed an inverse relationship between volume and in-hospital mortality, as detailed in **Tables 1** and **2**.

Table 1 In-hospital mortality based on hospital volume	
Total Hospital Volume, Annual Resections (N)	**In-hospital Mortality (%)**
<10	19
10–50	12
51–80	13
>80	6

Table 2	
In-hospital mortality based on surgeon volume	
Surgeon Volume, Annual Resections (N)	In-hospital Mortality (%)
<9	16
9–41	9
>41	5

Similar results were documented by Birkmeyer and colleagues,[4] who also showed that individual surgeon volume was inversely related to operative mortality for the Whipple procedure. Case volume should be included as a quality metric for pancreatic surgery not simply because of its strong correlation with mortality but also because it is easily measured and is likely a surrogate for other factors that influence surgical quality. In-depth systematic analyses of surgical techniques and perioperative management strategies that lead to improved outcomes are difficult to perform because of wide variability in practice among different hospitals and surgeons.

A high-volume pancreatic surgeon develops experience with preoperative planning and patient selection, develops an improved knowledge of anatomy and its variations, more astutely recognizes potential problems with perioperative care, and benefits from improvements in surgical technique that occur with frequent repetition. High-volume hospitals also develop infrastructure such as clinical pathways to guide postoperative care, multidisciplinary teams to discuss these cases in the preoperative and postoperative settings, and specialty services such as advanced interventional radiology or critical care teams. These various components nurture growth of the program and allow an institution's learning curve with this complex procedure to further develop.

ROLE FOR CENTRALIZATION OF PANCREATIC SURGERY

Centralization of pancreatic surgery in high-volume centers with better outcomes seems logical because pancreatic surgery is low volume and high risk compared with other types of elective surgical procedures. However, this approach may not be practical. Traveling to a high-volume center for a short period of time for surgery is more feasible than traveling repeatedly for chemotherapy or radiation. Preoperative imaging studies may also not be compatible from one institution to another and repeated work-up may lead to increased costs of care. However, advances in telemedicine may facilitate rapid sharing of information and allow streamlined communication between care facilities. For patients experiencing postoperative complications, long stays away from home can become burdensome. For these reasons and many more, centralization may not always be possible.

Studies on centralization of pancreatic surgery have thus far shown overall improvements in outcomes. A recent study from Canada described the effects of an explicit attempt by Canadian authorities to regionalize pancreatic resection in the province of Ontario. Beginning in 1999, Cancer Care Ontario initiated a series of quality improvement initiatives to limit pancreatic resection to hospitals performing 10 or more procedures per year with an operative mortality of less than 5%.[5] This initiative resulted in increased concentration of care, reflected by an increase in the median number of cases performed at hospitals meeting the baseline criteria and a reduction in the number of hospitals performing pancreatic resection.[5] Operative mortality also decreased in Ontario, from 8.7% in 1999 to 3.3% in 2000.[5] The investigators concluded that such a drastic reduction in only a year could be attributed to centralization of practice.

Although there is no mandate in the United States, studies documenting improved perioperative mortality with increasing volume, or perhaps other factors, seem to be leading to increasing centralization of pancreatectomy at high-volume centers. Stitzenberg and Meropol[6] reviewed a total of 17,658 pancreas cases documented between 1999 and 2007 in the Nationwide Inpatient Sample database, which weighs data to allow the estimation of population-level statistics. They showed a decrease in the total number of hospitals performing pancreas procedures over the study period and a statistically significant increase in high-volume centers from 38 in 1999 to 101 in 2008 (P = .003) (**Figs. 1** and **2**).[6] The proportion of procedures performed at low-volume centers also decreased over the study period. The likelihood of treatment of pancreatic cancer at a low-volume center in 2007 was significantly less than in 1999, with an odds ratio of 0.40 (95% confidence interval, 0.35, 0.46).[6]

TRAINING HIGH-QUALITY PANCREATIC SURGEONS

A learning curve exists for the Whipple procedure, which is one of the most technically intricate abdominal operations. Adding further complexity to the operation, it is typically performed on older patients with multiple comorbidities. Furthermore, as laparoscopic surgery evolves, minimally invasive pancreatic resections may be performed at gradually increasing rates, and using this new technology will have its own learning curve.

The finding that surgeons with higher volumes have improved outcomes suggests the presence of a learning curve for the Whipple procedure. Several reports have documented the learning curve for pancreaticoduodenectomy, with improvements in measurable quality metrics such as reduced estimated blood loss, operative times, and lengths of stay being shown over time.[7,8] However, it seems that near 100

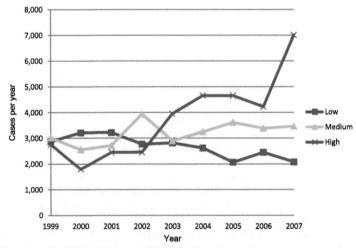

Fig. 1. Estimate of United States case volumes for pancreatic resections between 1999 and 2007. Volume category: low, 1 to 6 cases/y; medium, 7 to 26 cases/h; high, more than 26 cases/y. (*Data from* Stitzenberg KB, Meropol NJ. Trends in centralization of cancer surgery. Ann Surg Oncol 2010;17:2824–31.)

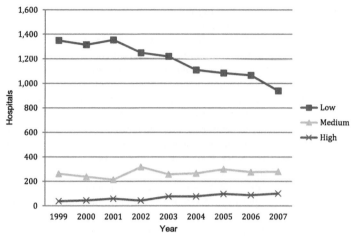

Fig. 2. Estimate of number of US hospitals of low, medium, and high volume between 1999 and 2007. Volume category: low, 1 to 6 cases/y; medium, 7 to 26 cases/h; high, more than 26 cases/y. (*Data from* Stitzenberg KB, Meropol NJ. Trends in centralization of cancer surgery. Ann Surg Oncol 2010;17:2824–31.)

pancreaticoduodenectomies may be required to reach proficiency, and analysis of additional cases beyond this landmark suggests that the learning curve continues further into a surgeon's career.[7]

According to the Accreditation Council for Graduate Medical Education, graduating US surgical residents in 2009 performed an average of only 5.6 (standard deviation, 5) pancreaticoduodenectomies during their training.[9] This is not enough experience or volume on which to begin a career of independent practice in pancreatic surgery and, therefore, most aspiring pancreatic surgeons require additional fellowship training. Furthermore, it may be critical to seek an environment with experienced colleagues and mentors who are willing to share their referral base. Centralization within the field inherently encourages selective referral to those with higher volumes, and, unless trainees are in an environment of high volume, they may not independently accrue sufficient cases because of lack of experience and referral bias.

There are currently 19 accredited fellowships in hepatopancreatobiliary surgery in the United States that will train almost 200 new pancreatic surgeons in the next 10 years. How this supply fares against the demand for pancreatic surgery remains unclear. With the aging of the population, the number of new pancreatic cancer cases in the United States has been projected to increase by 55% between 2010 and 2030.[10] This trend may increase the demand for pancreatic surgery in the years to come. The widespread use of diagnostic imaging has also resulted in more incidentally discovered pancreatic lesions, but understanding of the malignant potential of these lesions is progressing and more conservative approaches may prevail.

MORTALITY: A COMMON QUALITY METRIC AFTER PANCREATECTOMY

Mortality is one of the most easily obtained and reliable quality metrics. The first successful pancreaticoduodenectomy was performed in 1909 in Germany by Kausch[11] and reported in 1912. In 1935, Whipple and colleagues[12] reported a series of 3 patients of whom 2 survived the operation. By the end of Whipple's career, he had performed 37 pancreaticoduodenectomies.[13] Few surgeons attempted the procedure in the 1960s and 1970s because of a hospital mortality in the range of 25%. However, in the 1980s and 1990s, experience increased and reports from high-volume centers of operative mortality less than 5% began to appear in the literature.[14–16]

The improvement in operative mortality in the last 40 years is not only the result of increased technical experience but also of improved understanding of pancreatic disorders, advances in diagnostic radiology and medicine, meticulous preoperative planning, improved perioperative care, and (perhaps most importantly) the ability of modern hospital systems to address a wide array of postoperative complications through critical care, subspecialty, and interventional radiology services. As previously discussed, volume and mortality have repeatedly shown an inverse relationship. Birkmeyer and colleagues[4] postulated that more than 100 deaths in Medicare patients could be averted annually if pancreaticoduodenectomy were performed at high-volume centers, and suggested that, for patients who are considering pancreaticoduodenectomy at low-volume centers, the option of referral to a higher volume center should at least be made.

Operative mortality is easily and commonly measured. The target benchmark for mortality following pancreaticoduodenectomy is currently 5% or less per year. Institutions close to the border of high volume (around 20 pancreaticoduodenectomies per year) can therefore only experience 1 death annually if they are to compare with higher volume centers.

THE COMPLEXITY OF MEASURING QUALITY IN PANCREATIC SURGERY

Adequate case volumes have been associated with achieving safe pancreatic resections, but achieving high volume may not necessarily guarantee quality outcomes. Other quality metrics are needed to assess patient satisfaction and ensure excellent outcomes. However, beyond volume and operative mortality, measurement of quality metrics becomes complicated. For example, the available literature on reporting of postoperative complications has many limitations. The relationship between complication severity and the number of complications for each patient and their cumulative effect on outcomes is frequently unable to be assessed. A detailed and standardized definition of complications and severity grading is also often lacking. Differences in definitions can result in large variations in reported complication rates. Also, the tenacity with which evidence for every complication is sought out and recorded is variable even among programs with prospective collection. These differences make it difficult to compare reports from different institutions.

Despite these nuances, pancreatic surgery programs should actively and regularly track their cases to monitor outcomes and benchmark their performance against themselves over time and against others in the field. In the process of tracking data, systematic assessment with attention paid to grading each complication in adherence to standardized definitions is encouraged.

COMMONLY USED GRADING SYSTEMS

There is no consensus within the surgical community on the best way to report surgical complications. In 2002, Martin and colleagues[17] published their evaluation of the surgical literature as it related to the reporting of complications by assessing various studies' compliance with 10 predetermined criteria. These included the presence of a defined method of accruing data, duration of follow-up, inclusion of outpatient information, clear definitions of complications measured, reporting of causes of death and a calculated mortality, reporting of total complications and a morbidity rate, the assessment of procedure-specific complications, the use of a severity grading system, data on length of stay, and inclusion of patient-specific risk factors in the analysis. Overall, their study revealed wide variability in the level of compliance with these criteria. The investigators concluded that the variability observed could be attributed to the lack of consistent or standardized definitions of various complications.

Within the past 2 decades, many grading systems have emerged and these systems continue to evolve. The Clavien-Dindo system, originally introduced in 1992, ranked complications by severity based on the intervention required for treatment, and differentiated 3 types of negative outcomes after surgery: complications, failures to cure, and sequelae.[18] This system has since been revised to a 5-scale graded classification system for severity. This revised version also focuses on the therapeutic consequences of the complication. For example, life-threatening complications requiring intermediate or intensive care management are differentiated from complications addressed on the ward. Complications that have potential for long-term disability are also differentiated. This classification system has gained acceptance in the literature and has since been systematically assessed in many fields of surgery.[19,20]

The Common Terminology Criteria for Adverse Events (CTCAE) version 4.0 is another classification system that was originally developed by the National Cancer Institute and is commonly used throughout the oncology community.[21] It divides adverse events by system organ class and classifies these events into 5 general categories based on severity (mild, moderate, severe, life-threatening or disabling, and associated with death). The latest version includes 26 organ systems and more than 600 types of complications.

Aside from general complication grading systems, unique systems for procedure-specific complications should be used when available. In pancreatic surgery, these complications include pancreatic or biliary fistula formation or leak and delayed gastric emptying. For pancreatic fistula formation, the International Study Group of Pancreatic Fistula (ISGPF)[22] provides a grading system and, for delayed gastric emptying, the International Study Group of Pancreatic Surgery (ISGPS) has developed a grading system.[23] Some procedure-specific systems can be translated to the general complication grading systems. In **Tables 3** and **4**, for example, the ISGPF and ISGPS systems are compared with the CTCAE to show a certain degree of translatability.

QUALITY OUTCOMES FROM VARIOUS HIGH-VOLUME CENTERS

Table 5 shows a compilation of published data on commonly measured outcomes selected from high-volume centers with rigorous data collection. These benchmarks have to be interpreted in the context of the multitude of nuances that exist. Because of variability in reporting the components of operative morbidity such as delayed gastric emptying, rates of pancreatic fistula formation or anastomotic leaks, intra-abdominal infections, or wound complications, detailed comparisons among institutions are difficult to make.

ONE INSTITUTION'S DETAILED EXPERIENCE WITH OUTCOMES ASSESSMENT

Like many others, our group has invested in an institutional review board–approved prospective, electronic, Web-based database that tracks data on patient demographics, clinical history, past medical history, family and social history, physical examination findings, diagnostic test results, therapeutic interventions, complications, pathologic data, and short-term and long-term outcomes including perioperative mortality (90-day as well as in-hospital mortality) and survival for all patients seen in our pancreas center.

Data are collected prospectively in modules on electronic case report forms at specified times: initial visit, operation, discharge from the hospital, office visits, and

Table 3
Comparison of pancreatic fistula grading systems: CTCAE versus ISPGF

CTCAE Grade	CTCAE Description	ISPGF Grade	ISPGF Description
Grade 1	Asymptomatic No interventions required	Grade A	Asymptomatic No interventions required
Grade 2	Symptomatic with altered gastrointestinal function No invasive procedures required	Grade B	Symptomatic with altered gastrointestinal function No invasive procedures required Delay in discharge or readmission possible
Grade 3	Severely altered gastrointestinal function Nutritional support or elective operative or interventional procedure required	Grade C	Symptomatic with severely altered gastrointestinal function Nutritional support or urgent/emergent operative or interventional procedure required
Grade 4	Life-threatening consequences Urgent operative or interventional procedure required		Hospital stay extended or discharge delayed Complications such as sepsis, organ dysfunction, or
Grade 5	Death		death may ensue

Abbreviation: ISGPF, International Study Group of Pancreatic Fistula.

long-term data at 3-month intervals. Specific definitions of data elements and grading of complications are embedded into electronic case report forms. All complications are individually graded by severity, using the CTCAE system or complication-specific systems. Data are entered into the database in real time by a trained data analyst under the supervision of the surgeons. All data are backed up by source documents and the accuracy of the data entered into the electronic database is periodically audited. This system requires an ongoing investment of approximately $60,000/y. **Tables 6–9** summarize cumulative data from our center with a consecutive series of 159 pancreaticoduodenectomies and 78 distal pancreatectomies over the last 5 years.

RECENT DEVELOPMENTS IN QUALITY METRICS FOR PANCREATIC SURGERY

Several national initiatives are underway to provide a variety of opportunities for pancreatic surgeons and hospitals to examine quality metrics for pancreatic cancer care and identify areas for improvement. In a recently released study surveying 106 pancreatic surgeons in North America, Kalish and colleagues[34] identified quality metrics thought to be important by experienced pancreatic surgeons. The quality metrics thought to be most important were:

- Perioperative mortality
- Rate and severity of complications
- Access to multidisciplinary care

Other factors ranked highly by the surgeons polled in this survey included:

- Incidence of postoperative hemorrhage
- Venous thromboembolism prophylaxis
- Access to adjuvant therapies

Table 4
Comparison of delayed gastric emptying grading systems: CTCAE versus ISGPS

CTCAE Grade	CTCAE Description	ISGPS Grade	ISGPS Description
Grade 1	Mild nausea, early satiety and bloating, able to maintain caloric intake on a regular diet	Grade A	Nasogastric tube required between POD4 and POD7 or reinsertion because of nausea/vomiting after POD3 Inability to tolerate solid diet by POD7 but tolerates such by POD14 Symptoms or use of prokinetic agents may or may not be required
Grade 2	Moderate symptoms Able to maintain nutrition with dietary and lifestyle modifications May require pharmacologic intervention	Grade B	NGT required between POD8 and POD14 or reinsertion because of symptoms after POD7 Inability to tolerate solid diet by POD14 but tolerates such by POD21 Vomiting, gastric distention present, pharmacologic intervention required
Grade 3	Weight loss, refractory to medical intervention, unable to maintain nutrition orally Pharmacologic intervention required	Grade C	NGT required between POD14-21 or reinsertion caused by/because of symptoms after POD14 Inability to tolerate solid diet by POD21 Vomiting, gastric distention present, pharmacologic intervention required

Abbreviation: POD, post-operative day.

- Readmission rates
- Incidence of postoperative fistulas
- Timely and appropriate perioperative antibiotics
- One-year and 5-year survival rates
- Timing from diagnosis to surgical consultation

Bilimoria and colleagues[35] have also developed and tested quality indicators for pancreatic cancer using a formal methodology. They identified candidate quality indicators from the literature, current practice guidelines, and expert interviews. A multidisciplinary panel of pancreatic cancer experts ranked the potential quality metrics after 2 separate rounds of discussion. Analysis of rankings facilitated the development of a set of variables with high and moderate validity. An adapted version of their compiled list is presented later.

PANCREATIC CANCER QUALITY METRICS

Hospital responsibilities[35]:
- Require all pancreatic surgeons to be certified by the American Board of Surgery (or equivalent)

Table 5
Various quality measures from selected high-volume pancreas centers

	Mortality (%)[a]	Morbidity (%)	LOS (d)	Reoperation (%)	Or Time (min)	EBL (mL)
Pancreaticoduodenectomy						
BCM	1	48	9	<1	452	529
Hopkins[14]	1	41	9	3	330	700
Mayo[24]	NR	NR	12	7	401	1032
MGH[25]	1.7	37	12	2	NR	NR
UCSF[26]	4	59	16	7	402	1167
Virginia Mason[27]	<1	NR	11	<1	450	382
Laparoscopic Pancreaticoduodenectomy						
Pittsburgh[28]	2	30	10	6	568	350
Open Distal Pancreatectomy						
BCM	<1	42	8	0	260	440
Hopkins[14]	<1	31	10	6	258	450
Mayo[29]	1	25	8.6	NR	208	519
MSKCC[30]	<1	40	7	NR	163	350
Laparoscopic Distal Pancreatectomy						
BCM	<1	20	9	0	278	130
Emory[31]	<1	43	2.3	6	156	197
Mayo[29]	3	34	6.1	NR	214	171
MSKCC[30]	<1	27	5	NR	194	150
Pittsburgh[32]	1	50	7	NR	372	150
WashU[33]	0	32	4.5	4.5	236	244

Abbreviations: BCM, Baylor College of Medicine; EBL, estimated blood loss; LOS, length of stay; MGH, Massachusetts General Hospital; MSKCC, Memorial Sloan-Kettering Cancer Center; NR, not recorded; OR, operating room; UCSF, University of California San Francisco; WashU, Washington University in St Louis.

[a] Mortality measured at 30 days.

- Maintain 12 or more Whipples in the hospital and monitor individual pancreatic surgeon case volume
- Provide interventional radiology services, such as readily available on-site endoscopic retrograde cholangiopancreatography and endoscopic ultrasound capabilities, and an intensive care unit staffed by critical care physicians and specialists
- Monitor the R0 resection rate
- Maintain a risk-adjusted perioperative mortality of less than 5%
- Monitor median estimated operative blood loss, operative times (should be <10 hours), 30-day readmission rates, and stage-specific 2-year and 5-year survival rates for patients who undergo resection

Surgeon responsibilities:
- Provide thorough preoperative risk assessment for every case
- Perform accurate preoperative staging using high-quality imaging with triple-phase computed tomography or magnetic resonance imaging

Table 6
Patient characteristics, comorbid conditions, preoperative tests, and presenting signs and symptoms

	PD (n=159)	DP (n=78)
Patient Characteristics		
Age (y)	63 ± 12.5	59 ± 13
Gender (%)		
Male	76 (48)	34 (44)
Female	83 (52)	44 (56)
Race (%)		
White	127 (80)	65 (84)
African American	22 (14)	8 (10)
Asian	5 (3)	3 (4)
Pacific Islander	5(3)	2 (2)
Ethnicity (%)		
Hispanic	25 (16)	5 (7)
Comorbid Conditions and Preoperative Tests		
HTN	90 (57)	37 (49)
Diabetes	32 (20)	17 (22)
Chronic pancreatitis	22 (14)	8 (10)
CAD	20 (13)	8 (11)
COPD	8 (5)	6 (8)
Renal insufficiency	8 (5)	2 (3)
Obesity (BMI >30)	17 (11)	15 (20)
Smoking		
Current	28 (18)	13 (17)
Ever	38 (24)	20 (26)
Alcohol use		
Current	59 (37)	28 (36)
Ever	23 (15)	16 (21)
Total bilirubin	1.9 ± 3.4	0.3 ± 0.3
Creatinine	0.9 ± 0.4	1.0 ± 0.2
Albumin	4 ± 0.6	4.3 ± 0.6
Hemoglobin	13 ± 1.8	13 ± 1.7
Presenting Signs and Symptoms		
Anorexia	17 (11)	2 (3)
Constipation	2 (1)	5 (6)
Diarrhea	21 (13)	8 (10)
Early satiety	9 (6)	7 (9)
Jaundice	76 (48)	0 (0)
Nausea	50 (31)	18 (23)
Diabetes[a]	16 (10)	5 (7)
Pain	95 (60)	48 (62)
Vomiting	28 (18)	8 (10)
Weight loss	80 (50)	18 (23)

All values expressed as n (%) or value ± standard deviation.
Abbreviations: CAD, coronary artery disease; COPD, chronic obstructive pulmonary disease; DP, distal pancreatectomy; HTN, hypertension; PD, pancreaticoduodenectomy.
[a] Diabetes defined as new onset or recent exacerbation (within 2 years before diagnosis of pancreatic disease).

Table 7 Intraoperative data and pathologic diagnoses		
	PD	**DP**
Intraoperative Details		
OR time (min)	452 ± 99	266 ± 88
EBL (mL)	529 ± 638	374 ± 400
PD size (mm)	4.4 ± 2.2	2.5 ± 1.6
Soft pancreas	91 (57)	47 (60)
PD stent placement	74 (47)	1 (1)
Vein resection	27 (17)	1 (1)
Transfusion	27 (17)	4 (5)
Pathologic Diagnoses		
Adenocarcinoma	86 (54)	18 (23)
Pancreatic	58 (36)	16 (20)
Ampullary	24 (15)	0 (0)
Other	4 (3)	2 (3)
Neuroendocrine	12 (7)	14 (19)
Cystic neoplasm	32 (20)	37 (47)
IPMN	23 (14)	10 (13)
MCN	4 (3)	15 (19)
Cystadenoma	5 (3)	8 (10)
Pseudopapillary	0 (0)	4 (5)
Pancreatitis	6 (4)	2 (2)
Adenoma	6 (4)	1 (1)
Other	17 (11)	6 (8)
Total	159 (100)	78 (100)

All values expressed as n (%) or value ± standard deviation.
Abbreviations: IPMN, intraductal papillary mucinous neoplasm; MCN, mucinous cystic neoplasm.

- Document the absence of regional arterial involvement, metastatic disease, and distant adenopathy (suspicious adenopathy outside the resection or liver, omental, or peritoneal lesions should be submitted for frozen section)
- Document the removal of all pancreatic tissue, lymph nodes, and connective tissue between the edge of the uncinate process and the right lateral wall of the superior mesenteric artery for patients undergoing pancreaticoduodenectomy

Responsibilities of the multidisciplinary team:
- Provide multidisciplinary care (including the services of a surgical, medical, and radiation oncologist) for every patient
- Record clinical and pathologic stage for each patient and devise a stage-specific treatment plan
- Provide resection for patients with stage I or II disease or document a valid reason for not undergoing resection
- Perform surgery or provide first nonsurgical treatment within 2 months from the time of diagnosis
- Provide adjuvant chemotherapy with or without radiation therapy or document a valid reason for not doing so and note the timing of initiation of such treatments in relation to surgery

Table 8
Pathologic staging of resected pancreatic adenocarcinomas

	PD (n=58)	DP (n=16)
Tumor size	3.2 ± 1.2	4.0 ± 2.6
Lymph Nodes		
Number examined	23 ± 8.5	18.3 ± 9.7
Number positive	4.4 ± 4.8	1.8 ± 2.5
Tumor Stage		
Stage 0	0	0
Stage IA	3 (5)	1 (6)
Stage IB	2 (3)	0 (0)
Stage IIA	8 (14)	7 (44)
Stage IIB	45 (78)	8 (50)
Histologic Grade		
G1 (well differentiated)	4 (7)	2 (13)
G2 (moderately differentiated)	29 (50)	9 (56)
G3 (poorly differentiated)	25 (43)	5 (31)
Lymphovascular invasion	37 (64)	2 (13)
Perineural invasion	47 (81)	3 (19)
Resection Margin Status		
R0	43 (74)	14 (88)
R1	13 (23)	1 (6)
R2	2 (3)	1 (6)

All values expressed as n (%) or value ± standard deviation.

- Provide chemotherapy or chemoradiation for patients who do not undergo surgical resection or document a valid reason for not providing nonsurgical therapy
- Provide opportunities for patients to participate in clinical trials

Responsibilities of pathology:
- Maintain adherence to the College of American Pathologists checklist or an equivalent reporting system
- Document the histology, grade, tumor size, margin status, number of lymph nodes excised (should be ≥10), number of lymph nodes involved, and tumor-node-metastasis stage for all patients who undergo resection

The Commission on Cancer of the American College of Surgeons (ACS) and the American Cancer Society have developed the National Cancer Data Base (NCDB), a nationwide oncology outcomes database for more than 1500 accredited cancer programs in the United States. This database provides hospitals with reports regarding their performance on various process measures.[36] The database will soon add outcome measures for 30-day mortality and 5-year survival for pancreatic cancer. Thus, hospitals will be able to evaluate themselves in comparison with the other approximately 1000 hospitals that perform pancreatic surgery.

Although the Commission on Cancer offers some information on pancreatic surgery processes of care, limited data are currently available on postoperative complications. This situation may also soon change with the ACS National Surgical Quality Improvement Program (NSQIP) pilot program examining surgical cancer care, ACS NSQIP

Table 9
Ninety-day complication rates

	PD	DP
Patients with any complication ≥ grade I or grade A[a]	70 (44)	33 (42)
Patients with any complication ≥ grade II or grade B	39 (25)	16 (20)
Patients with any complication ≥ grade III or grade C	24 (15)	9 (12)
Mean severity grade of complications[b]	2	2
Patients with 1 complication	42 (26)	20 (26)
Patients with 2 complications	13 (8.2)	9 (11)
Patients with 3 complications	7 (4.4)	3 (3.8)
Patients with 4 complications	2 (1.3)	0 (0)
Patients with ≥ 5 complications	2 (1.3)	2 (2.5)
Specific Complications		
ARDS	1 (<1)	0 (0)
Biliary leak	1 (<1)	0 (0)
Death	1 (<1)	0 (0)
Gastroparesis[c]	15 (9.4)	3 (3.8)
Grade A	9 (5.7)	3 (3.8)
Grade B	4 (2.5)	0 (0)
Grade C	2 (1.2)	0 (0)
Hepatic failure	0 (0)	0 (0)
Intra-abdominal abscess	8 (5.0)	6 (7.7)
Severity grade 2	1 (<1)	1 (1.3)
Severity grade 3	7 (4.4)	5 (6.4)
Myocardial infarction	2 (<1)	0 (0)
Pancreatic fistula[d]	36 (22)	17 (22)
Grade A	16 (10)	9 (12)
Grade B	12 (7.5)	4 (5)
Grade C	8 (5.0)	4 (5)
Pneumonia	1 (<1)	1 (1.3)
Postoperative hemorrhage	1 (<1)	0 (0)
Reoperation	1 (<1)	0 (0)
Readmission	13 (8.1)	19 (24)
Renal failure	2 (1.2)	0 (0)
Urinary tract infection	4 (2.5)	4 (5.1)
Venous thromboembolism	5 (3.1)	1 (1.3)
Severity grade 2	3 (1.9)	0 (0)
Severity grade 3	2 (1.3)	1 (1.3)

(continued on next page)

Table 9 (continued)		
	PD	DP
Wound infection	10 (6.3)	5 (6.4)
Severity grade 2	4 (2.5)	1 (1.3)
Severity grade 3	6 (3.8)	4 (5.1)
Wound dehiscence	0 (0)	1 (1.3)

All values shown as n (%).
Abbreviation: ARDS, acute respiratory distress syndrome.
[a] Complications were graded in severity using the CTCAE (v4.0) (grade 1–5), unless otherwise specified.
[b] Complications with grades A, B, and C were converted to 1, 2, and 3 respectively to calculate median complication severity scores.
[c] Gastroparesis was graded using the ISGPS definition.[23]
[d] Pancreatic fistula was graded using the ISGPF definition.[22]

Oncology.[37] Pancreatic cancer is a component of this project. Participating institutions provide patient data, such as demographics, comorbid conditions, laboratory values, clinical characteristics, and operative variables. They prospectively follow patients for 30 days postoperatively, tabulating various postoperative complications, such as surgical site infections, urinary tract infections, pneumonias, renal failure, venous thromboembolic events, unplanned intubations, reintubations, and readmissions.[32] Risk-adjusted 30-day morbidity and mortality outcomes are computed for each participating hospital and made available semiannually to provide participating hospitals with performance data comparisons with other institutions.

SUMMARY

Few established quality metrics in pancreatic surgery exist. Many published institutional experiences provide a general idea of the state of pancreatic surgery and share a set of potential benchmarks against which other surgeons can assess themselves, but they collectively show variability. As the practice of pancreatic surgery evolves to encompass a wider array of clinical indications and incorporate increasingly complex technologies, systematic assessment of quality and outcomes is imperative. It has been repeatedly shown that outcomes are superior when pancreaticoduodenectomy is performed by high-volume surgeons practicing in hospitals with a high caseload. As a result, centralization of pancreatic surgery has resulted in a decrease in the total number of hospitals performing pancreas procedures over time and an increase in the number of high-volume pancreas centers. These centers should continue to provide high-quality training for future pancreatic surgeons and support progression along the learning curve that exists for pancreatic surgery. Several national initiatives are underway to provide new opportunities for pancreatic surgeons and hospitals to examine quality metrics for pancreatic cancer care and identify areas for improvement.

REFERENCES

1. Bilimoria KY. Advancing the quality of pancreatic cancer care. National Quality Measures Clearinghouse. Available at: http://www.qualitymeasures.ahrq.gov/expert/printView.aspx?id=36833. Accessed October 10, 2012.

2. Rosales-Velderrain A, Stauffer JA, Bowers SP, et al. Current status of laparoscopic distal pancreatectomy. Minerva Gastroenterol Dietol 2012;58:239–52.
3. Lieberman MD, Kilburn H, Lindsey M, et al. Relation of perioperative deaths to hospital volume among patients undergoing pancreatic resections for malignancy. Ann Surg 1995;222:638–45.
4. Birkmeyer JD, Finlayson SR, Tosteson AN, et al. Effect of hospital volume on in-hospital mortality with pancreaticoduodenectomy. Surgery 1999;125:250–6.
5. Sonnenday CJ, Birkmeyer JD. A tale of two provinces: regionalization of pancreatic surgery in Ontario and Quebec. Ann Surg Oncol 2010;17:2535–6.
6. Stitzenberg KB, Meropol NJ. Trends in centralization of cancer surgery. Ann Surg Oncol 2010;17:2824–31.
7. Tseng JF, Pisters PW, Lee JE, et al. The learning curve in pancreatic surgery. Surgery 2007;141:694–701.
8. Fisher WE, Hodges SE, Wu MF, et al. Assessment of the learning curve for pancreaticoduodenectomy. Am J Surg 2012;203:684–90.
9. Hardacre JM. Is there a learning curve for pancreaticoduodenectomy after fellowship training? HPB Surg 2010;2010:230287.
10. Smith BD, Smith GL, Hurria A, et al. Future of cancer incidence in the United States: burdens upon an aging, changing nation. J Clin Oncol 2009;27: 2758–65.
11. Kausch W. Das carcinoma der papilla duodeni und seine radikale entfeinung. Beitr Z Clin Chir 1912;78:439–86.
12. Whipple A, Parsons WB, Mullins CR. Treatment of carcinoma of the ampulla of Vater. Ann Surg 1935;102:763–79.
13. Whipple AO. A reminiscence: pancreaticoduodenectomy. Rev Surg 1963;20: 221–5.
14. Cameron JL, Riall TS, Coleman J, et al. One thousand consecutive pancreaticoduodenectomies. Ann Surg 2006;244:10–5.
15. Winter JM, Cameron JL, Campbell KA, et al. 1423 Pancreaticoduodenectomies for pancreatic cancer: a single-institution experience. J Gastrointest Surg 2006; 10:1199–211.
16. Cameron JL, Pitt JA, Yeo CJ, et al. One hundred and forty-five consecutive pancreaticoduodenectomies without mortality. Ann Surg 1993;217:430–8.
17. Martin RC, Brennan MF, Jaques DP. Quality of complication reporting in the surgical literature. Ann Surg 2002;235(6):803–12.
18. Clavien PA, Sanabria JR, Strasberg SM. Proposed classification of complications of surgery with examples of utility in cholecystectomy. Surgery 1992;111: 518–26.
19. Dindo D, Demartines N, Clavian PA. Classification of surgical complications: a new proposal with evaluation in a cohort of 6336 patients and results of a surgery. Ann Surg 2004;240:205–13.
20. Clavien PA, Barkun J, de Oliveira ML, et al. The Clavien-Dindo classification of surgical complications: five year experience. Ann Surg 2009;250(2):187–96.
21. US Department of Health and Human Services. Common terminology criteria for adverse events (CTCAE) version 4.03. Available at: http://evs.nci.nih.gov/ftp1/CTCAE/About.html. Accessed October 3, 2012.
22. Bassi C, Dervenis C, Butturini G, et al. Postoperative pancreatic fistula: an International Study Group (ISGPF) definition. Surgery 2005;138:8–13.
23. Wente MN, Bassi C, Dervenis C, et al. Delayed gastric emptying (DGE) after pancreatic surgery: a suggested definition by the International Study Group of Pancreatic Surgery (ISGPS). Surgery 2007;142:761–8.

24. Asbun HJ, Stauffer JA. Laparoscopic vs open pancreaticoduodenectomy: overall outcomes and severity of complications using the Accordion severity grading system. J Am Coll Surg 2012;215:810–9.
25. Balcom JH, Rattner DW, Warshaw AL, et al. Ten year experience with 733 pancreatic resections: changing indications, older patients, and decreasing length of hospitalization. Arch Surg 2001;136:391–8.
26. Schell MT, Barcia A, Spitzer AL, et al. Pancreaticoduodenectomy: volume is not associated with outcome within an academic health care system. HPB Surg 2008;2008:825940.
27. Traverso LW, Shinchi H, Low DE. Useful benchmarks to evaluate outcomes after esophagectomy and pancreaticoduodenectomy. Am J Surg 2004;187:604–8.
28. Zeh HJ, Zureikat AH, Secrest A, et al. Outcomes after robot-assisted pancreaticoduodenectomy for periampullary lesions. Ann Surg Oncol 2012;19:864–70.
29. Vijan SS, Ahmed KA, Harmsen WS, et al. Laparoscopic vs open distal pancreatectomy: a single institution comparative study. Arch Surg 2010;145:616–21.
30. Jayaraman S, Gonen M, Brennan MF, et al. Laparoscopic distal pancreatectomy: evolution of technique at single institution. J Am Coll Surg 2010;211:503–9.
31. Kneuertz JP, Patel SH, Chu CK, et al. Laparoscopic distal pancreatectomy. J Am Coll Surg 2012;215:167–76.
32. Daouadi M, Zureikat AH, Zenati MS, et al. Robot-assisted minimally invasive distal pancreatectomy is superior to the laparoscopic technique. Ann Surg 2013;257:128–32.
33. Pierce RA, Spitler JA, Hawkins WG, et al. Outcomes analysis of laparoscopic resection of pancreatic neoplasms. Surg Endosc 2007;21:579–86.
34. Kalish BT, Vollmer CM, Tseng JF, et al. Advancing quality assessment in pancreatic surgery: defining the role of the Institute of Medicine healthcare quality domains. 46th Annual Meeting of the Pancreas Club. San Diego, May 18–19, 2012.
35. Bilimoria KY, Bentrem DJ, Lillemoe KD, et al. Assessment of pancreatic cancer care in the United States based on formally developed quality indicators. J Natl Cancer Inst 2009;101:848–59.
36. Bilimoria KY, Stewart AK, Winchester DP, et al. The National Cancer Data Base: a powerful initiative to improve cancer care in the United States. Ann Surg Oncol 2008;15:683–90.
37. Bilimoria K, Wang X, Cohen ME, et al. Development of ACS NSQIP Oncology: A Surgical Quality Measurement System for cancer centers paper presented at Society of Surgical Oncology Annual Meeting. San Antonio, March 2–5, 2011.

The Economics of Pancreas Surgery

Charles M. Vollmer Jr, MD

KEYWORDS

- Economics • Costs • Pancreatic resection • Clinical pathway • Complications

KEY POINTS

- Care must be taken when comparing surgical cost-analysis studies given the myriad cost-accounting techniques used. Intrastudy cost comparisons are far more relevant than are interstudy assessments.
- Clinical care pathways for pancreatic surgery have demonstrated not only a clinical benefit to patients but also considerable resource conservation.
- Cost assessments are increasingly becoming useful outcome metrics, allowing for comparisons of the technical variations of pancreatic surgical care beyond traditional clinical parameters.
- Complications and readmissions contribute significantly to the overall cost of pancreatic surgery.
- Pancreas surgery is a paramount example of the impact that regionalization of care can have on cost savings.
- The economics of surgery can be assessed at numerous echelons, from the granular (patient) level through to the global (societal) perspective.

INTRODUCTION: NATURE OF THE PROBLEM

The age of medical superspecialization is on us. Although this era has brought us significant progress in patient outcomes, it also coincides with the most explosive period of health-cost inflation. Heretofore, the cost of care was of negligible concern to practicing physicians. Now, one of the principle dilemmas in medicine is cost containment. For surgery, no procedure represents specialization better than pancreatic resection given the high acuity of the patients, the operative prowess required of the surgeon, and the significant reliance on advanced and constantly evolving technologies. Because it has been a model for noteworthy clinical outcomes research, pancreas surgery has, not surprisingly, also offered numerous contributions to our understanding of health care economics. These contributions span many echelons of analysis, from

Department of Surgery, Hospital of the University of Pennsylvania, University of Pennsylvania School of Medicine, 3400 Spruce Street, 4th Floor, Silverstein Pavilion, Philadelphia, PA 19104, USA
E-mail address: Charles.Vollmer@uphs.upenn.edu

Surg Clin N Am 93 (2013) 711–728
http://dx.doi.org/10.1016/j.suc.2013.02.010
0039-6109/13/$ – see front matter © 2013 Elsevier Inc. All rights reserved.

granular (patient care) to global (societal). This article appraises the current knowledge base of pancreatic surgery economics and reveals novel, emerging concepts that promise to impact the delivery of care to our patients in the future.

THE LEXICON OF HEALTH CARE ECONOMICS

It is important to understand that there is no codified language used across the cost analyses presented in the literature. No two reports seemingly offer comparable objective data. Therefore, it is very difficult to discern variation between studies. Depending on institutional accounting and reporting preferences, studies reveal a plethora of cost structures, few of which are equivalent. In some cases, cost descriptions reflect extended time periods beyond the patients' index hospitalization and may also include readmission costs. Furthermore, for data accrued over protracted time frames, some reports incorporate adjustments for inflation (using the medical component of the consumer price index [CPI]). Probably more valuable are *intrastudy* comparisons or ratios. Also relevant to this discussion is the fact that although statistically significant differences may not be seen when cost is used as a metric, there is still an effect in real dollars saved or lost, which may have a considerable fiscal consequence.

The following list provides a general framework of definitions to help interpret the literature on surgical health care economics.

Charges

Charges are an amount of money for care that patients or a third-party payer is *asked to* pay by the provider. Charges represent a claim made to insurance payers that is commonly inflated 2 to 3 times more than the expected reimbursement. Thus, charges are relatively abstract and largely irrelevant.

Costs

Cost is a general term that reflects the *actual price required* to provide the medical service rendered. Costs may vary considerably geographically. For instance, the price of a sequential compression device or a particular surgical stapling device is not globally equal. Being more concrete than charges, costs are not as influenced by the biases of different payer's profit margins.

Direct Costs

Direct costs are expenses directly related to the provision of care for a specific patient. If the service did not occur, there would be no expense. This figure is the one most often presented in the literature because it is a tangible entity.

Indirect Costs

Indirect costs are expenses for running the hospital that are allocated to all patients but not directly related to a specific patient's care. For instance, a patient may be charged a certain fraction of the global maintenance costs (lighting, new equipment, and so forth) of a particular ward. A different interpretation of this definition may be the costs to society, beyond the hospital setting, such as lost worker productivity. Naturally, because of its collective nature, the specific accounting of this category is imprecise and, therefore, it is ignored in most patient-centered cost calculations.

Itemized Costs

Itemized costs are a breakdown of the various components of surgical care. Often these are referred to as *cost centers* for direct costs. For instance, a surgical patient accrues charges from the operating room, the pharmacy, the blood bank, the floor, the intensive care unit (ICU), and so forth.

Total Costs

Properly defined, this is an aggregate of direct and indirect costs. However, be careful in reading the literature because most studies place qualifiers. For instance, many articles obviate the contribution of indirect costs given how nebulous their accounting can be. Furthermore, the summation of itemized components is not generally consistent between studies.

Professional Fees

Professional fees are the fees charged by the practitioner for compensation of their specific contributions to care. These fees generally adhere to the current procedural terminology (CPT) coding process whereby services are assigned prices within a specific framework. Professional fees are *rarely* integrated into the literature reports on costs given that they are usually derived from separate accounting systems than those that the hospital uses for cost and charge assessment.

Reimbursement/Revenue

Reimbursement and *revenue* are interchangeable words that represent the actual amount of money received from the payer for services provided by either the hospital or the physician. This amount is usually a significant fraction of the charges, yet can be modestly higher than costs.

Contribution Margin

Contribution margin is the revenue minus the direct costs, otherwise referred to as the *gross profit*.

Net Gain or Loss

Net gain or *net loss* is the contribution margin with the additional subtraction of the indirect component of costs, also recognized as *net profit* or *net loss*.

The reader is urged to scrutinize the methods section of each study presented herein to make appropriate judgments of the findings.

COST AND THE CONCEPT OF QUALITY
What is the Cost of Pancreatectomy?

One of the earliest descriptions of the cost of major pancreatectomy came in 1996. With the specter of managed care emerging, Holbrook and colleagues[1] developed some of the first notions of concept of *value* in surgery by using pancreaticoduodenectomy (PD) as a paradigm for major surgery.[1] Cost data from 30 PDs performed from 1993 to 1995 were prospectively accrued in aggregate and also itemized. The mean overall cost was $17 252, 21% of which represented operating room expenditures. It was also the first report of the direct association of postoperative complications on increased resource utilization and, therefore, cost (see later discussion). There was no difference between PDs performed for malignancy and for benign conditions. Their conclusion was that by scrutinizing drivers of cost, surgeons could better implement changes that would improve quality.

Systems Improvements and Cost

Although the ensuing decade brought a handful of articles that described the cost basis of major pancreatectomy (presented later in this article), a more contemporary assessment of benchmark outcomes in pancreatic resection surgery, including the total cost of care, was described in 2007.[2] This work described how improvements in delivery of care for close to 300 major pancreatectomies correlated with cost containment. Over a 5-year period, the total cost of care per patient decreased significantly from $31 541 to $18 829. The effect was more profound with PD than with distal resections. This finding correlated strongly with a concurrent decrease in the observed-to-expected (O/E) ratio of complications over the same period, attributed largely to the implementation of a clinical care path. The investigators suggested that each 10% improvement in performance (O/E) equates to roughly a $2500 cost savings per patient. Laboratory, pharmacy, and radiology cost centers had the most relevant impact on cost savings.

Does Surgical Performance Influence Cost?

The same specialty group from the Beth Israel Deaconess Medical Center (BIDMC) in Boston extended their analysis of variables, which lead to better outcomes following pancreatectomy by focusing on the concept of operative performance.[3] Using the physiologic and operative severity score for the enumeration of mortality and morbidity (POSSUM) system, the interplay between patients' baseline physiology and operative conduct was explored. Costs (and other outcomes) decreased up to 14% with patients' improved physiologic function. Similarly, optimal intraoperative performance was associated with lower rates of morbidity, length of stay (LOS), and cost (up to a 17% decrease). Patients with the worst physiology and a suboptimal operation cost $23 087, whereas the other end of the spectrum (lowest acuity with best operative performance) cost more than $6000 less. The single most influential driver of surgical performance in this construct was blood loss. The investigators showed that each additional unit (375 mL) of blood loss cost an additional $4000 per patient. Analogously, in terms of patient acuity, each 10-year increase in patient age was associated with a $3000 cost increase.

The Price of Aging

With increased scrutiny on the appropriation of health care resources, the controversial notion of rationing continues to percolate. Restriction of operations by age occurs worldwide for some surgical procedures. It is, therefore, important to define the appropriate value for pancreatectomy for the elderly to determine if it is a wasteful expenditure. Pratt and colleagues[4] established benchmark outcomes for pancreatectomy in the elderly (defined as patients aged 75 years or older), a cohort accounting for one-fifth of their resections. In a highly specialized pancreatic surgical practice with a focused process for care of elderly patients, they were able to show overall clinical outcomes on par with younger patients. Despite the obvious higher patient acuity, the cost of care was delivered for $19 852 per elderly, a marginal 12% increase of $2200 more than younger patients. Further detailing revealed that minor and moderate deviations of care were no more debilitating on elderly patients. Yet, when major deviations occurred, they had a significant impact on outcomes and cost; the cost of care for those elderly patients who had major deviations was $45 000 more than the similar scenario in a younger patient. As a consequence, when adjusting for the impact of complications on patient outcomes, elderly patients actually cost greater than $9000 ($\approx$33%) more per case.

THE IMPACT OF CLINICAL CARE PATHS ON THE COST OF PANCREATECTOMY

The application of clinical care paths to complex HPB surgery was first described by Pitt and colleagues[5] who showed improvements in outcomes as well as significant cost savings (measured by hospital *charges*) in biliary bypass surgery in the 1990s. They concluded that the introduction of care paths, and feedback from the results obtained, was an effective method to control costs in the academic medical center setting.

Conventional Pathway Analyses

Naturally, it did not take long for this process to be applied to pancreatic resection surgery. The group from MD Anderson Cancer Center provided the first such model.[6] Over 3 years, 68 PDs were compared with 80 PDs after a pathway was implemented. The mean total costs were reduced by almost a quarter, from $47 515 to $36 627; this followed suit with a decreased LOS by 3 days. Notably, other major outcomes (mortality, readmissions, and so forth) did not vary because of the pathway. The greatest reductions were evident in room and board, diagnostics, nutrition, and other postoperative care costs. Multivariate analysis revealed the pathway status to be independently associated with total costs. The costs reported in this series included physician costs, a rare presentation in the cost literature, yet did not include indirect costs. The take-home point from this study is that behaviors dictated by a structured pathway can positively influence resource utilization, even if clinical outcomes are largely unaffected.

Another series of reports on the implementation of clinical pathways for major pancreatectomy ensued from the group at Thomas Jefferson University. They describe significant improvements in hospital stay and cost metrics (*charges* in this case) when a multidisciplinary pathway was introduced for PD.[7] The hospital duration dropped by 6 days (almost half), and average charges decreased an astounding 47% ($240 000 to $127 000). In a separate report, they reported analogous findings for distal pancreatectomy.[8] In that case, hospital readmissions were significantly decreased (25% decreased to 7%) and hospital *costs* decreased by $3500, although this was not statistically significant. It should be noted, however, that the outcome differences occurred in conjunction with a virtually new pancreatic specialty group at that institution (resulting in a 4-fold increase in volume in a short period), so there may be confounders as to why such dramatic improvements occurred.

Deviation-Based Cost Modeling

Pathways have reproducibly demonstrated improvements in diminishing LOS and the use of hospital resources, albeit without reducing actual complication occurrence. They seem to provide a framework for identifying waste of resources. What remains curious is whether the gains are caused by the pathway explicitly or caused by secular changes (naturally occurring improvements) in care over time. Secondly, it is not certain if pathways can successfully mitigate the impact of postoperative complications. To attack these concerns, the group from BIDMC described a novel quality-assessment approach, which relies on weighted-mean averaging of the contribution of deviations from the expected pathway (deviation-based cost modeling).[9] Deviations refer to a combination of complications and LOS and reflect when patients are *off pathway*.

The clinical and economic outcomes of 209 PDs from 2001 to 2006 were described in the setting of the implementation of a unique clinical pathway (64 before and 145 after). Overall, a $3551 savings per patient was evident by traditional pathway analysis. Although this did not reach statistical significance, it did represent an absolute decrease in costs of 15%. More patients remained on course with the use of the pathway, largely because of fewer *minor* deviations in care. Total costs differed significantly for all categories of deviations after the pathway. As deviations became more pronounced, so did costs. Weighted average mean cost was used to more accurately measure cost efficiency. This approach showed that the overall cost savings per patient was more like $5542. From this, pathway-dependent costs were derived and found to be equivalent to secular costs ($2780 vs $2762, respectively).

THE FINANCIAL BURDEN OF COMPLICATIONS
Complications Following Pancreatic Resection: Frequent and Costly

Outcomes for high-acuity surgery have been highly scrutinized over the last decade with the maturation of large administrative datasets and increased sophistication in biostatistical methodology. Initial concentrations focused on the ultimate outcome metric following surgery, mortality, which is a highly impactful yet relatively rare occurrence. Subsequently, concentration has turned to understanding complication rates, which are far more common and are perhaps the most realistic surrogate for quality of care. Interestingly, cases of mortality, although devastating personally and emotionally, are not usually the most costly economically. Conversely, complications (particularly major complications) are particularly resource avid and, therefore, expensive. A significant evaluation of national outcomes for pancreatectomy using the National Inpatient Sample (NIS) database defined that complications occurred 23% of the time and were independent predictors of death, prolonged hospital stay, and discharge to another facility. Although mortality rates have steadily declined temporally, complication rates have remained static. The investigators intimated, but did not explicitly show, that these findings must have a profound effect on health care costs.[10] As mentioned earlier, Holbrook and colleagues[1] initially demonstrated this to be true at the practice level in the 1990s.

Enestvedt and colleagues[11] showed that complications nearly doubled the cost of care after 145 PDs performed in a network of community-based teaching hospitals during a contemporary time frame (2005–2009). Only direct costs for the index hospitalization and readmissions were considered; physician's fees were not. The overall complication rate was 69%, but major complications occurred in 26% of the patients. They suggested that the clustering of numerous other complications with major complications contributed greatly to the heightened costs of a complicated case (ie, a derivative effect is seen). The median cost for PD was $30 937 but differed significantly (P<.001) for the presence of major complications ($56 224 with vs $29 038 without). Multivariate analysis demonstrated the following complications to have a significant impact on costs: reoperation, delayed gastric emptying, pancreatic fistula, bile leak, pulmonary, renal, and thrombotic events, as well as sepsis. Furthermore, certain cost centers contributed greatly to the additive costs of complications; for instance, pharmacy costs increased an average of $26 334 when complications occurred.

In a nice comparative study, Clavien's group from Switzerland investigated the economic impact of complications associated with 1200 major abdominal operations, including 110 major pancreatic operations, performed within the same hospital.[12] They used their own well-recognized and validated complication scoring scale to dissect the costs associated with these procedures[13] and used a standardized national cost accounting system. For the overall cohort, mean costs increased dramatically with the severity of the complication: $28 000 for uncomplicated grade 0 cases versus $159 000 for grade IV complications (life-threatening events requiring ICU management). The magnitude of the increase was most impressive with pancreatic resections as compared with the other procedures. They showed that the cost of a death was significantly higher than grades I to III complications, but much lower than grade IV cases (P<.001). For all the operations studied, the cost of care was most expensive for pancreas resection cases ($71 111 vs $45 924 for the overall series) but was equivalent for those cases without any complications ($31 809).

Pancreatectomies with complications cost $16 000, $20 000, and $47 000 more than complicated colorectal resections, liver surgeries, or Roux-en-Y gastric bypasses, respectively. This article was the first to show that the costs associated with similarly severe complications can vary by type of surgery, and the investigators suggest that this provides evidence that reimbursement for procedures should be adjusted for the complication risk profile of the particular procedure.

Another group has recently looked at the impact of complications on compensation within the confines of the German reimbursement model.[14] In a limited analysis of 36 patients, they showed that complications doubled duration of hospital stay (16 vs 33 days) and increased costs, particularly for ICU treatment and radiographic diagnostics. For 21 patients without any complications, it cost €10 015, whereas it averaged €15 340 for the 15 patients with complications. However, compensation based on the German Diagnostic Related Group's (DRG) scales yielded payments of €13 835 and €15 062, respectively. This finding indicates a positive balance for noncomplicated cases and a slight deficit for complicated cases. The investigators argue that these realities indicate that cost neutrality can only be achieved in those centers that demonstrate lower complication rates and go so far as to suggest that this objective is best achieved in high-volume specialty centers.

The Costs of Specific Postpancreatectomy Complications

Infections
Infection control has recently come to the forefront as a quality measure for hospitals and practitioners. In some cases, compensation is being withheld in such scenarios with the implication that infectious morbidity should be preventable. For an example, of complex gastrointestinal surgery, the group from BIDMC probed the burden of infectious complications following 550 major pancreatic resections and included a cost analysis that included readmissions.[15] Infectious complications occurred in 31% of the resections, with wound infections and infected pancreatic fistulas happening most frequently. The total costs were, on average, $15 000 more expensive for cases with infections; this accounted for 40% of the cost differential, grade for grade. The most costly impact was for the grade IV category ($\approx$$80 000), reflecting a 5-fold cost differential over noninfected cases. They note that the true economic impact is likely underestimated because postdischarge dispositions were not accounted for.

Pancreatic fistulas
Postoperative pancreatic fistulas (POPFs) are referred to as the Achilles heel of pancreatic resections. Pratt and colleagues,[16] who used costs as a distinct outcome metric to validate a newly conceived definition scheme for fistulas, investigated the price of POPFs following PD. Using the proposed International Study Group of Pancreatic Fistula scale, the investigators were able to show increasing expenses (along with numerous clinical parameters) as POPFs progressively escalated from no fistula across 3 POPF severity grades. Economically, grade A (transient, biochemical leaks) patients are no different from patients who lack complications ($18 075 vs $18 209, $P = .68$). Furthermore, as the fistula severity increased from grade A to C, all total and itemized cost metrics correspondingly escalated to the point where grade C fistulas cost an astounding $119 083 per patient (43% of this attributed to ICU boarding). Other resource utilization was extreme for patients who developed grade C fistulas. Combined radiology, pharmacy, laboratory, and transfusion costs alone ($19 680) rival overall hospital costs for grade A ($18 075) POPFs.

The same group also showed similar findings for POPFs following distal and central pancreatectomies but identified how those fistulas differ clinically and economically from those after PD.[17] Again, for each resection type, costs progressively escalated across the various severity grades. Grade B fistulas were more expensive for distal resections ($34 555) when compared with PDs ($27 778), whereas the cost of treating grade C fistulas was far less expensive (by almost $100 000). On the other hand, the economic profile of POPFs after central resections was analogous to that of proximal resections. This article used the cost of care as a relevant metric to help establish differences in the severity and behavior of fistulas that occur following the spectrum of pancreatic resections. Another report suggests that POPFs following distal pancreatectomies (33% frequency in 66 patients) contribute to a doubling of mean costs when compared with those patients who do not leak.[18] Using a decision-analysis model, they suggested that any hypothetical intervention to reduce the fistula rate following distal pancreatectomy (DP) by a clinically realistic one-third would be justified if it cost less than $1400 per patient.

The Predicament of Readmissions

The topic of readmissions is currently in the vanguard, especially as regulatory agencies and payers increasingly seem to equate readmission to a mark of initially failed care. Furthermore, the financial impact of readmissions on the health care system is not trivial; thus, readmission rates have become a hot outcome metric. Readmission following high-acuity abdominal surgery is common, occurring in roughly one-fifth of the cases. Reasons for readmission following major pancreatectomy include treatment of complications; inadequate nutrition (failure to thrive); and, in many cases, just to investigate complaints that do not manifest as overt problems. The first clinical analysis of this for pancreatectomy occurred at the national level using the Surveillance Epidemiology and End Result (SEER) database (1730 Medicare patients, 1992–2003).[19] Readmission rates were 16% at 30 days and 53% at 1 year. Early readmissions were dominated by complication management (80%), but the rest were caused by unrelated diagnoses. Late admissions, by contrast, were caused by recurrence of the disease half the time. Other studies of PD have ensued, with similar conclusions.[20,21]

Although these studies introduced us to the scope of the clinical issues, the economic realities of this problem were still poorly elucidated because of the nature of the databases used. Kent and colleagues[22] probed the financial implications of readmissions on pancreatic surgical care in their single-institution practice at BIDMC. Nineteen percent of the 578 patients who had major pancreatectomies were readmitted. The costs of *index* hospitalization was more than $6000 higher in readmitted patients, which is not surprising because complications encountered during the original hospitalization are strongly associated with readmission. The typical cost of a readmission event (median LOS = 7 days) was an additional $10 000. Therefore, the $16 000 additive cost incurred by readmitted patients equated to 164% of the overall cost of care for nonreadmitted patients. The investigators make 2 important points. First, the true costs are underestimated because certain factors, such as initial evaluations at other facilities, transport costs, postdischarge nursing and rehabilitation resources, and physicians' fees, were not accounted for in their analysis. Second, if these rates and costs are representative, readmissions might account for $500 000 per annum in each high-volume specialty surgical practice.

FISCAL ANALYSIS OF VARIOUS TECHNIQUES IN PANCREATIC SURGERY
Is Minimally Invasive DP Cheaper?

The 2000s have marked an era of the extension of minimally invasive surgery (MIS) from simple surgical procedures to advanced technical endeavors in solid organ surgery.

For various reasons, the pancreas has been the final frontier for this innovation. None-theless, there has been a considerable advance toward performing major pancreatec-tomy through either laparoscopic or, more recently, robotic means. Although there has not yet been a comparative analysis of the cost of performing MIS PD, headway has been made in understanding the economic implications of MIS DP.

Four series, from 3 different countries, have recently assessed the laparoscopic DP for its cost-effectiveness. Abu Hilal and colleagues[23] from the United Kingdom reviewed 51 DPs performed from 2005 to 2011 whereby clinical outcomes were essentially equivalent. They compared direct costs of the operative intervention, the postoperative recovery period (including readmission), as well as a conglomerate of total costs for both open (n = 16) and laparoscopic (n = 35) operations. Intraoperative costs were significantly higher, whereas postoperative costs were considerably less when DP was performed laparoscopically. Although the additive effect was a nonsig-nificant difference in total costs (both with and without readmissions considered), the laparoscopic technique seemed considerably cheaper (around £5400 or 32%). The in-vestigators posited that these differences are only going to become more accentuated as technical prowess with the laparoscopic approach continues to be refined. A very similar series from Italy, albeit with muted cost discrepancies between the two tech-niques, came to the same conclusions.[24]

A more robust series emanates from the specialty Hepato-Pancreato-Biliary (HPB) unit in Toronto, which conforms to the single-payer, publically funded Canadian health care system.[25] Indirect costs, but not personal compensations, were accounted for in their methodology; costs were adjusted for inflation to 2010 Canadian dollars. From 2004 to 2010, 118 DPs were performed (42 laparoscopically). The hospital duration of stay was significantly lower (5 vs 7 days) by laparoscopy, but all other major quality outcomes were equivalent, including operating room time. Preoperative and intrao-perative (surprisingly) costs did not differ, yet open DP resulted in significantly higher costs in all other hospital departments (recovery room, imaging, laboratories, and pharmaceuticals) as well as total costs (median $2800 more expensive). They also re-ported that LOS was a significant predictor of all cost domains (exclusive of preoper-ative and operative costs), whereas complications were not.

Although the preceding 3 articles describe single-institution experiences that relied on detailed, local cost accounting, a more global assessment of the employment of MIS DP throughout the United States was conducted, which called on the NIS, SEER, and National Surgical Quality Improvement Program (NSQIP) administrative da-tabases.[26] Laparoscopy was used for only a fifth of all cases reported. Complications, duration of stay, and costs were less when laparoscopy was used. Median expenses were reported to be $44 741 for laparoscopy and $49 792 for open resections (P = .02). Caution should be used when interpreting these figures. First, it is unclear from the article's methodology whether this represents charges or costs but probably the former. Second, the figures are subject to myriad inaccuracies common to national administrative database analysis. The investigators concluded that centralization of this procedure to academic specialty units was *not* occurring.

Finally, yet another competitive technology has emerged for pancreatic resection. The group from Indiana University reported their initial, yet significant (77 DPs in 1 year), experience with robotic DP.[27] Seventeen robotic DPs were compared with 28 laparoscopic and 32 open cases. Spleen preservation was achieved far more often (65%) with robotic DP, but they also took close to an hour longer. Surprisingly, robotic DP was the cheapest technique (total direct costs: $10 588 vs $16 059 open and $12 986 laparoscopic). Likely, this was driven by significant, parallel differences in postoperative duration of stay. No mention is made of the acquisition cost and overhead for the robot. They concluded that robotic DP is a safe and cost-effective technique in selected cases.

Comparison of Parenchymal Sparing and Radical Pancreatic Resections

Controversy exists regarding whether some patients can derive clinical benefit from parenchymal sparing resections for certain pancreatic pathologic conditions The balance is between the negative effects of short-term complications (primarily leaks) on one side and long-term exocrine and endocrine insufficiencies on the other. The pancreatic specialty unit in Verona has a rich experience with managing these scenarios. They report an experience of 21 parenchymal-sparing operations and 64 DPs for cases of benign neoplasia in the body and tail of the pancreas over the 1990s.[28] Early postoperative clinical outcomes favored distal pancreatectomy, yet costs (as determined by procedural DRG) were equivalent for cases without complications (€2890 for central pancreatectomy vs €3181 for DP). However, when complications did occur, parenchymal-preserving techniques were considerably more expensive (by 32%). They proposed that middle pancreatic resection is suboptimal given its higher complication and cost profiles. However, the long-term costs of increased rates of diabetes and steatorrhea in the DP group were not accounted for.

Comparison of Operations for Chronic Pancreatitis

Numerous options are available for the treatment of chronic pancreatitis, including nonoperative versus operative approaches or various techniques when operations are chosen. Chronic pancreatitis is a cost-avid, protracted, debilitating disease with significant implications to societal resource utilization. Howard and colleagues[29] reported the clinical and economic effectiveness of surgical management using either duodenum-preserving (Beger procedure) or traditional (PD) resection options. Both techniques showed equivalent and significant improvements of clinical outcomes and costs for a period of 1 year after surgery when compared with nonoperative management the year preceding. Direct hospital and physician costs were considered in this study, and figures were adjusted to 1996 dollars based on the medical CPI. PD was slightly more expensive in terms of hospital costs than was duodenum-preserving resection ($25 746 vs $21 878, $P = .489$). However, these figures increased even more, becoming statistically significant when physician costs were factored in. More importantly, the average yearly disease-specific hospital-based costs decreased after surgery by more than 50% for both techniques, indicating the effectiveness of surgery for managing this disease process. Cost outlays were shown to shift from symptom management to treating complications incurred by surgery. These findings have been corroborated by a similar investigation from Japan, which showed that patients who required endoscopic-based therapies for longer than a year had higher medical expenses than patients who were treated with surgery.[30]

The Cost-effectiveness of Octreotide Therapy

The clinical value of octreotide therapy for preventing pancreatic fistulas after PD is well studied, yet remains controversial worldwide. Two articles, with different analytical approaches, have assessed the economic value of this therapeutic adjunct.

Rosenberg and colleagues[31] created an elaborate *theoretical* decision-tree analysis whereby costs were estimated and assigned to each branch of the tree depending on its clinical outcome. In their first derivation, average per diem hospitalization direct costs (around $552 per day) were obtained from Statistics Canada for an estimated LOS. Patients with pancreatic fistulas were estimated to be hospitalized an additional 21 days longer. This finding suggested that in a cohort of 100 patients, 16 would avoid complications at an average cost savings of $853 per patient if octreotide was used. However, in a second derivation whereby costs were acquired from the Ontario Case Costing Project, that savings effect doubled. This cost basis was derived by a more modern approach of summation of average detailed cost centers required for postoperative care. However, the costs used did not link directly to any particular patient because the model was completely speculative. They concluded, "Since the rate of occurrence of fistula is relatively low, it is difficult to justify the use of octreotide in all patients. However, in patients at risk for developing a complication, its administration is a cost-effective strategy."[31]

Recognition that distinct risk factors exist for the development of pancreatic fistulas after PD in the current era of the International Study Group for Pancreatic Fistula (ISGPF) definition[32] allowed the BIDMC group to test that same notion.[33] Using an actual patient care experience of 227 consecutive PDs performed from 2001 to 2007, total hospital costs were compared between those patients who actually received prophylactic octreotide (56%) against those who did not. When stratified for the presence of risk factors for fistulas, the investigators found that the administration of octreotide in low-risk scenarios had no clinical benefit and was cost-ineffective ($781 loss per patient, approximately the cost of a 7-day course of the drug). Conversely, in high-risk patients, octreotide decreased fistula rates and led to decreased resource use, affording a cost savings of almost $12 000 per high-risk patient. Similar to the last article, the investigators advocated its use only in high-risk cases to achieve maximal benefit.

The Price of Medical versus Surgical Palliation of Unresectable Pancreatic Cancer

A report from the Mayo Clinic in the 1990s was among the first to indicate that endoscopic biliary drainage of unresectable pancreatic cancer may rival surgical palliation.[34] Despite the need for multiple endoscopic procedures (mean 1.7 stent changes at $1190 each), equivalent survival was realized at a lower cost and shorter hospital stay.

Is Staging Laparoscopy for Pancreatic Malignancy Cost-effective?

With the advent of MIS and alternative palliation techniques in the late 1990s, staging laparoscopy emerged as a useful clinical tool for eliminating unnecessary laparotomies for unresectable pancreatic cancer.[35] Despite clear-cut clinical data supporting its use, cost-effectiveness data are limited. Part of the dilemma is the multiple possible branches of the palliative algorithm in these patients. Holzman and colleagues[36] established that, for unresectable tumors, the cost of palliation performed at the time of laparoscopy was a third cheaper than palliation at the time of open exploration ($9700 vs $14 500). However, procedures converted from laparoscopic to open were far more costly at $20 100. General trends across the literature reveal that intraoperative costs are higher for laparoscopic cases, yet the lower overall cost structure for these cases is the result of dramatically decreased hospital durations. To be more cost-effective, it has been suggested that the yield of laparoscopic staging needs to be as high as 30%, which is a level of efficiency encountered initially but rarely today when the yield is closer to 10%.[37]

In a more contemporary look at this question, Enestvedt and colleagues[38] linked primary medical record data to a population-based cancer registry to calculate the economic impact from across the state of Oregon. In a unique approach, average hospital and physician charges were derived from a single institution and then applied to a malleable clinical performance model accrued from statewide practice patterns. The charges for routine, case-specific, or nonuse of staging laparoscopy were equivalent ($91 805, $90 888, $93 134, respectively). They concluded that neither routine nor selective use of laparoscopy added significant costs to the overall care of potentially resectable pancreatic cancer.

Does It Pay to Follow Up Pancreatic Cancer Surgery?

A recent investigation has looked into the economics of surveillance for the recurrence of pancreatic cancer after a successful resection operation.[39] Patterns of care for post-resection abdominal imaging were examined from 1991 to 2005 using Medicare's SEER database. Over the time period studied, the median number of computed tomography scans obtained doubled. Univariate analysis of those patients with the best survival outcomes demonstrated that there was no defined benefit to annual imaging. Costs were estimated using Medicare Part-B line-item reimbursement. For the 11 850 studies performed on 2217 patients, costs per patient for this surveillance were roughly $1400 (as high as $1800 in 2005). However, this was thought to be an extremely conservative estimate. The investigators suggested that, through this analysis, the cost-effectiveness, as well as the putative oncologic benefit, of repeated axial imaging is to be questioned.

THE MACROECONOMICS OF PANCREATIC SURGERY
The Volume-Outcomes Story

Warshaw,[40] recognizing the impending onset of managed care in the 1990s, editorialized that pancreatic surgery represents a model for surgical centralization that would likely result in more economic delivery of care. Significant inroads to the implications of this prediction have been made over the last 2 decades.

Influence of the institution

Since the landmark article by Birkmeyer in 2002, the association of procedural volume to outcomes has been scrutinized for many operations.[41] That article showed that, for all of the high-risk operations studied, the largest gains in decreasing mortality risk occurred when pancreatectomy was performed by high-volume institutions (a 4-fold decline over low-volume institutions). A follow-up article reports the effect this original work has had on the regionalization of major operations a decade later and shows that 67% of the decrease in mortality for pancreatectomy is a consequence of higher hospital volume.[42] Still curious is the influence of the surgeon on outcomes improvement in pancreatic surgery as well as the impact of regionalization on the cost of care.

Predating Birkmeyer's work was a seminal report that showed the potential effect regionalization might have for major pancreatectomy. In this work, Gordon and colleagues[43] described the differential results achieved between high- and low-volume institutions in the state of Maryland in the 1990s. In essence, this compared the outcomes at a single high-volume regional institution (Johns Hopkins) against collective outcomes of 38 other hospitals (each low volume). Although profound differences were seen in mortality and LOS at the regional center, when adjusted for other confounding variables, hospital charges were about one-fifth less for all discharges ($5011, P<.001). Over the time course of the study, charges dropped considerably at the regional hospital and they increased at the other hospitals. The investigators estimated that 17% of the total cost of care for pancreatectomy in the state could have been eliminated if the cases performed at the low-volume institutions were instead directed to the regional center.

In a related follow-up report, the same investigators studied the effects of institutional volume on other components of pancreatic cancer care. Although clinical outcomes were again clearly superior for curative surgical resection, palliative surgical bypasses, and endoscopic stenting at the high-volume center, they did not find similar trends in cost savings.[44] Only pancreatectomy was found to be significantly cost-efficient, underscoring the uniqueness of this particular endeavor.

Contemporaneous reports from other large state data registries substantiate these findings.[45,46] However, appreciating that most PDs are still performed in community hospitals, this is a contentious issue that may significantly impact physician commerce and livelihood. In a retort to the Gordon article, one surgeon from Maryland indicated that equivalent outcomes and costs could be achieved at community hospitals.[47] However, an interesting article by Chappel and colleagues[48] looked at the effects that the regionalization of complex operations would have on the bottom line of small hospitals. Charges from 14 rural hospitals in New York State were converted to revenue estimates for abdominal aneurysm repair, carotid endarterectomy, colectomy, cystectomy, esophagectomy, and pancreatectomy. Collectively these operations provided just more than 2% of the annual revenue of these hospitals. Most of this was provided by colectomies (1.93%), whereas the others *combined* accounted for just 0.16%. The effect of pancreatectomy was negligible because only 6 cases were performed in 3 years in these select hospitals. They argued that the transfer of pancreatectomy to regional specialty centers would not challenge hospital viability.

The individual surgeon's role in cost containment
These findings regarding institutional effects on costs have been controversial; perhaps surgeons themselves can drive cost reduction? A study from an academic community medical center in Portland suggests that they can.[49] In a single institution, a high-volume pancreatic surgeon (>10 per year) demonstrated markedly better mortality and morbidity outcomes than 15 other low-volume surgeons. The median costs were again shown to be $5820 less (a common figure throughout this review), although this was not statistically significant. Only a higher American Society of Anesthetists (ASA) level was predictive of costs. Itemized pharmacy charges (total parenteral nutrition, antibiotics, and octreotide) contributed the most and likely represent a surrogate marker for more complications in the low-volume cohort.

This perspective is substantiated by another report that instead used administrative discharge data derived from 266 648 patients across 3 states. Here the investigators compared the relative contributions to costs between hospital and surgeon factors for 6 cancer operations, including pancreatectomy.[50] Costs were derived by converting charges using certain cost-to-charge ratios and then adjusting for inflation. Lower costs were clearly associated with higher surgeon volume for all 6 procedures, but only colectomy was associated with higher hospital volume. Costs for the delivery of care continued to decline for all procedures over the 11 years studied (1989–2000). Again, it was found that high-volume surgeons perform PD for $5935 (about one-fifth) less than low-volume surgeons. They suggested that cost savings are best achieved through surgeon-specific referrals.

Local Economics

What is the value of pancreatic surgery to a hospital?
A high-volume specialty unit in pancreatic surgery can be a valuable asset to a health care system's viability, whereas occasional performance of these procedures is not (as discussed earlier). Given the prominent case-mix index of these patients, as well as relatively generous weighting of DRGs for pancreatic conditions, compensation for pancreatic surgical care is significant. As some basic reference points, in 2011, the average hospital reimbursements for PD and DP are on the order of $ 42 000 and $35 000, respectively. In contrast, a surgeon's professional compensations for the same procedures are around $3300 and $2000. These figures are generic

estimates and may vary widely given fluctuations in local reimbursement contracting. As an example of the effect at the practice level, the author's own pancreatic specialty surgical group at the University of Pennsylvania (2 surgeons, ≈1000 patient encounters, and 150 major pancreatic resections per annum) accounts for a contribution margin of more than $6 million and, when indirect costs are accounted for, a net gain of close to $2 million each year. More importantly, each pancreatic surgical patient has a considerable derivative effect on the system, beyond the confines of the surgery department, in that numerous ancillary services are required (intensive care, radiology, anesthesia, and so forth) to achieve optimal outcomes. Furthermore, proper multidisciplinary care often engenders downstream services from other major hospital departments, such as medical and radiology oncology; thus, there is a mushroom effect to each patient treated. Collectively, HPB patients provide an average of more than a $22 000 contribution per discharge, 1.5 times that for other surgical procedures performed in the author's system.

Societal Economics

Does insurance status affect surgical care?

Numerous reports have emerged over the last decade indicating discrepancies in surgical care of underprivileged patients. Using the National Cancer Data Base and logistic regression analysis, Bilimoria and colleagues[51] provided a provocative look at reasons why patients with resectable (stage 1) pancreatic cancer either refused or were not offered surgery. Among other variables, patients were less likely to undergo surgery if their insurance was either Medicare or Medicaid or they had lower annual incomes.[51] Similarly, primary payer status has been found to predict early mortality and survival after major surgical procedures.[52] This study, using NIS data, also showed that Medicaid and uninsured patients had longer durations of stay and total costs. This last point is intriguing, suggesting that less optimal insurance is associated with more expensive care. Although these articles do not directly deal with the costs of care, they provide an alternative fiscal perspective by suggesting that people who do not hold private insurance ultimately suffer worse service and outcomes.

Is pancreatic surgery a valuable use of resources?

Oncologic outcomes from pancreatic cancer surgery remain disappointing despite significant improvements in technical prowess and systems delivery that have mitigated morbidity and substantially reduced mortality over the last 40 years.[53] This realization, coupled with heightened concern for health care inflation, has led some to question the societal utility of treating this disease.[54] In a provocative meta-analysis, Gudjonsson[54] provided evidence of fewer *actual* long-term survivors than the literature suggests, claiming that many published series are duplicative. He estimated that only 1 in 30 patients who were resected with curative intent lived 5 years. At an estimated cost of $150 000 per resection, the proposed cumulative cost per successful resection is $4.5 million dollars. The implication was that resections for pancreatic cancer should be abandoned because of their minimal impact and considerable waste of resources. A counterpoint to this was provided by Gordon and Cameron[55] who brought into question the assumptions in the model used to establish these figures, particularly for deriving costs.

The cost utility of pancreatic cancer surgery

Experts in cost-effectiveness analysis have proposed that quality-adjusted life years (QALYs) become a standard metric for calibrating the value of health outcomes.[56,57] In essence, QALYs integrate health-related quality-of-life measures to convey health status in terms of equivalents of well years of life, which, in turn, can be associated with the cost of care. Using the total direct lifetime costs for treatments for pancreatic cancer surgery, Swedish investigators estimated the cost of a QALY to be €35 000.[58] Adams,[59] in an astute editorial, lauds this work as a benchmark for cost-utility analysis for pancreatic surgery, noting that these figures compare favorably with other accepted cancer therapies as well as to other chronic conditions like renal dialysis.

Theoretical Economics

Are costs reflective of quality?

Many consider *quality* to mean deriving good value from a product. By definition, *value* implies a quantitative comparison. As such, the cost of a service is often considered in calculating value and, therefore, quality. Recently, a survey was conducted among a collection of international pancreatic surgical specialists asking what outcomes measure *quality* care for pancreatic surgery.[60] Respondents were asked to rank more than 60 separate metrics in terms of relevance to surgical quality and then requested to align them with 6 Institute of Medicine (IOM) quality domains.[61] Traditional outcomes assessment measures, such as mortality, complications, and use of multidisciplinary care, ranked highest. Only 16% of the surgeons thought that the total cost of care was an *essential* domain, and all cost indicators ranked in the lower half of perceived importance. Metrics related to costs were found to align most often with the IOM domain of efficiency. The investigators suggested that this low importance professed by surgeons is incongruent with the heightened emphasis health care purchasers and policy makers are placing on cost assessments.

SUMMARY

There is a rich collection of literature reflecting the economic aspects of delivering pancreatic surgical care. Costs have been shown to fluctuate across numerous variations of the technical aspects of pancreatic surgery, both in and out of the operating room. Clinical care paths seem to reign in the cost of care by reducing waste. Pancreatectomy is a paradigm of regionalization of care whereby clinical outcomes are improved along with the benefit of cost reduction. Costs are emerging as a promising outcomes metric. However, the definitions and applications of this variable are far from codified. To be more meaningful, better standardization of health care economic outcomes definitions need to be established so that interstudy analyses can be more relevant. Nonetheless, pancreas surgery provides a good platform for continued endeavors in cost-effectiveness research.

REFERENCES

1. Holbrook RF, Hargrave K, Traverso LW. A prospective cost analysis of pancreaticoduodenectomy. Am J Surg 1996;171(5):508–11.
2. Vollmer CM, Pratt W, Vanounou T, et al. Quality assessment in high-acuity surgery: volume and mortality are not enough. Arch Surg 2007;142(4):371–80.
3. Pratt W, Callery MP, Vollmer CM. Optimal surgical performance attenuates physiologic risk in high-acuity operations. J Am Coll Surg 2008;207(5):717–30.
4. Pratt WB, Gangavati A, Agarwal K, et al. Establishing standards of quality for elderly patients undergoing pancreatic resection. Arch Surg 2009;144(10):950–6.
5. Pitt HA, Murray KP, Bowman HM, et al. Clinical pathway implementation improves outcomes for complex biliary surgery. Surgery 1999;126:751–8.
6. Porter GA, Pisters PW, Mansyur C, et al. Cost and utilization impact of a clinical pathway for patients undergoing pancreaticoduodenectomy. Ann Surg Oncol 2000;7(7):484–9.

7. Kennedy EP, Rosato EL, Sauter PK, et al. Initiation of a critical pathway for pancreaticoduodenectomy at an academic institution–the first step in multidisciplinary team building. J Am Coll Surg 2007;204(5):917–23.

8. Kennedy EP, Grenda TR, Sauter PK, et al. Implementation of a critical pathway for distal pancreatectomy at an academic institution. J Gastrointest Surg 2009;13(5): 938–44.

9. Vanounou T, Pratt W, Fischer JE, et al. Deviation-based cost modeling: a novel model to evaluate the clinical and economic impact of clinical pathways. J Am Coll Surg 2007;204:570–9.

10. Simons JP, Shah SA, Ng SC, et al. National complication rates after pancreatectomy: beyond mere mortality. J Gastrointest Surg 2009;13(10):1798–805.

11. Enestvedt CK, Diggs BS, Cassera MA, et al. Complications nearly double the cost of care after pancreaticoduodenectomy. Am J Surg 2012;204:332–8.

12. Vonlanthen R, Slankamenac K, Breitenstein S, et al. The impact of complications on costs of major surgical procedures: a cost analysis of 1200 patients. Ann Surg 2011;254(6):907–13.

13. Dindo D, Demartines N, Clavien PA. Classification of complications: a new proposal with evaluation in a cohort of 6336 patients and results of a survey. Ann Surg 2004;240:205–13.

14. Tittelbach-Helmrich D, Abegg L, Wellner U, et al. Insurance costs in pancreatic surgery: does the pecuniary aspect indicate formation of centers? Chirurg 2011;82(2):154–9 [in German].

15. Kent TS, Sachs TE, Callery MP, et al. The burden of infection for elective pancreatic resections. Surgery 2013;153(1):86–94.

16. Pratt W, Maithel SK, Vanounou T, et al. Clinical and economic validation of the International Study Group of Pancreatic Fistula (ISGPF) classification scheme. Ann Surg 2007;245(3):443–51.

17. Pratt W, Maithel SK, Vanounou T, et al. Postoperative pancreatic fistulas are not equivalent after proximal, distal and central pancreatectomy. J Gastrointest Surg 2006;10(9):1264–78.

18. Rodriguez JR, Germes SS, Pandharipande PV, et al. Implications and cost of pancreatic leak following distal pancreatic resection. Arch Surg 2006;141(4):361–5.

19. Reddy DM, Townsend CM, Kuo YF, et al. Readmission after pancreatectomy for pancreatic cancer in Medicare patients. J Gastrointest Surg 2009;13(11):1963–74.

20. Yermilov I, Bentrem D, Sekeris E, et al. Readmissions following pancreaticoduodenectomy for pancreas cancer: a population-based appraisal. Ann Surg Oncol 2009;16(3):554–61.

21. Ahmad SA, Edwards MJ, Sutton JM, et al. Factors influencing readmission after pancreaticoduodenectomy: a multi-institutional study of 1302 patients. Ann Surg 2012;256(3):529–37.

22. Kent TS, Sachs TE, Callery MP, et al. Readmission after major pancreatic resection: a necessary evil? Surgery 2011;213(4):515–23.

23. Abu Hilal M, Hamdan M, Di Fabio F, et al. Laparoscopic versus open distal pancreatectomy: a clinical and cost-effectiveness study. Surg Endosc 2012; 26(6):1670–4.

24. Limongelli P, Belli A, Russo G, et al. Laparoscopic and open surgical treatment of left-sided pancreatic lesions: clinical outcomes and cost-effectiveness analysis. Surg Endosc 2012;26(7):1830–6.

25. Fox AM, Pitzul K, Bhojani F, et al. Comparison of outcomes and costs between laparoscopic distal pancreatectomy and open resection at a single center. Surg Endosc 2012;26(5):1220–30.

26. Rosales-Velderrain A, Bowers SP, Goldberg RF, et al. National trends in resection of the distal pancreas. World J Gastroenterol 2012;18(32):4342–9.
27. Waters JA, Canal DF, Wiebke EA, et al. Robotic distal pancreatectomy: cost effective? Surgery 2010;148(4):814–23.
28. Falconi M, Mantovani W, Frigerio I, et al. Intermediate resection and distal pancreatectomy for benign neoplasms of the pancreas: comparison of postoperative complications and costs. Chir Ital 2001;53(4):467–74.
29. Howard TJ, Jones JW, Sherman S, et al. Impact of pancreatic head resection on direct medical costs in patients with chronic pancreatitis. Ann Surg 2001;234(5):661–7.
30. Hirota M, Asakura T, Kanno A, et al. Long-period pancreatic stenting for painful chronic calcified pancreatitis required higher medical costs and frequent hospitalizations compared with surgery. Pancreas 2011;40(6):946–50.
31. Rosenberg L, MacNeil P, Turcotte L. Economic evaluation of the use of octreotide for prevention of complications following pancreatic resection. J Gastrointest Surg 1999;3(3):225–32.
32. Pratt WP, Callery MP, Vollmer CM. Risk prediction for the development of pancreatic fistula using the ISGPF scheme. World J Surg 2008;32(3):419–28.
33. Vanounou T, Pratt WB, Callery MP, et al. Selective administration of prophylactic octreotide during pancreaticoduodenectomy: a clinical and cost-benefit analysis in low- and high-risk glands. J Am Coll Surg 2007;205(4):546–57.
34. Raikar GV, Melin MM, Ress A, et al. Cost-effective analysis of surgical palliation versus endoscopic stenting in the management of unresectable pancreatic cancer. Ann Surg Oncol 1996;3(5):470–5.
35. Stefanidis D, Grove KD, Schwesinger WH, et al. The current role of staging laparoscopy for adenocarcinoma of the pancreas: a review. Ann Oncol 2006;17:189–99.
36. Holzman MD, Reintgen KL, Tyler DS, et al. The role of laparoscopy in the management of suspected pancreatic and periampullary malignancies. J Gastrointest Surg 1997;1:236–44.
37. Obertop H, Gouma DJ. Essentials in biliopancreatic staging: a decision analysis. Ann Oncol 1999;10:150–2.
38. Enestvedt CK, Mayo SC, Diggs BS, et al. Diagnostic laparoscopy for patients with potentially resectable pancreatic adenocarcinoma: is it cost-effective in the current era? J Gastrointest Surg 2008;12(7):1177–84.
39. Witkowski ER, Smith JK, Ragulin-Coyne E, et al. Is it worth looking? Abdominal imaging after pancreatic cancer resection: a national study. J Gastrointest Surg 2012;16(1):121–8.
40. Warshaw AL. Pancreatic surgery – a paradigm for progress in the age of the bottom line. Arch Surg 1995;130:240–6.
41. Birkmeyer JD, Siewers AE, Finlayson EV, et al. Hospital volume and surgical mortality in the United States. N Engl J Med 2002;346:1128–37.
42. Finks JF, Osborne NH, Birkmeyer JD. Trends in hospital volume and operative mortality for high-risk surgery. N Engl J Med 2011;364(22):2128–37.
43. Gordon TA, Burleyson GP, Tielsch JM, et al. The effects of regionalization on cost and outcome for one general high-risk surgical procedure. Ann Surg 1995;221(1):43–9.
44. Sosa JA, Bowman HM, Gordon TA, et al. Importance of hospital volume in the overall management of pancreatic cancer. Ann Surg 1998;228(3):429–38.
45. Lieberman MD, Kilburn H, Lindsey M, et al. Relation of perioperative deaths to hospital volume among patients undergoing pancreatic resection for malignancy. Ann Surg 1995;222(5):638–45.

46. Glasgow RE, Mulvihill SJ. Hospital volume influences outcome in patients undergoing pancreatic resection for cancer. West J Med 1996;165(5):294–300.

47. Schaefer CJ. Cost and outcome of the Whipple procedure. Ann Surg 1995; 222(2):211–2.

48. Chappel AR, Zuckerman RS, Finlayson SR. Small rural hospitals and high-risk operations: how would regionalization affect surgical volume and hospital revenue? J Am Coll Surg 2006;203:599–604.

49. Kennedy TJ, Cassera MA, Wolf R, et al. Surgeon volume versus morbidity and cost in patients undergoing pancreaticoduodenectomy in an academic community medical center. J Gastrointest Surg 2010;14(12):1990–6.

50. Ho V, Aloia T. Hospital volume, surgeon volume, and patient costs for cancer surgery. Med Care 2008;46(7):718–25.

51. Bilimoria KY, Bentrem DJ, Ko CY, et al. National failure to operate on early stage pancreatic cancer. Ann Surg 2007;246(2):173–80.

52. LaPar DJ, Bhamidipati CM, Mery CM, et al. Primary payer status affects mortality for major surgical operations. Ann Surg 2010;252(3):544–50.

53. Lewis RS, Drebin JA, Callery MP, et al. A contemporary analysis of survival for resected pancreatic ductal adenocarcinoma. HPB (Oxford) 2013;15(1):49–60.

54. Gudjonsson B. Carcinoma of the pancreas: critical analysis of costs, results of resections, and the need for standardized reporting. J Am Coll Surg 1995;181(6): 483–503.

55. Gordon TA, Cameron JL. Management of patients with carcinoma of the pancreas. J Am Coll Surg 1995;181:558–60.

56. Weinstein MC, Seigel JE, Gold MR, et al. Recommendations of the panel on cost-effectiveness in health and medicine. JAMA 1996;276:1253–68.

57. Weinstein MC, Skinner JA. Comparative effectiveness and health care spending – implications for reform. N Engl J Med 2010;362:460–5.

58. Ljungman D, Lundholm K, Hyltander A. Cost-utility estimation of surgical treatment of pancreatic carcinoma aimed at cure. World J Surg 2011;35(3):662–70.

59. Adams DB. Life, liberty and the pursuit of quality-adjusted life years after pancreatic cancer surgery. World J Surg 2011;35(3):473–4.

60. Kalish BT, Vollmer CM, Kent TS, et al. Quality assessment in pancreatic surgery: what might tomorrow require? J Gastrointest Surg 2013;17(1):86–93.

61. National Institute of Medicine. Crossing the quality chasm: a new health system for the 21st century. National Academies Press; 2001.

Index

Note: Page numbers of article titles are in **boldface** type.

Surg Clin N Am 93 (2013) 729–739
http://dx.doi.org/10.1016/S0039-6109(13)00048-0
0039-6109/13/$ – see front matter © 2013 Elsevier Inc. All rights reserved.

surgical.theclinics.com

Printed and bound by CPI Group (UK) Ltd, Croydon, CR0 4YY

03/10/2024

01040442-0017